WOMEN'S PROGRESS
Promises and Problems

WOMEN IN CONTEXT: Development and Stresses

BECOMING FEMALE: PERSPECTIVES ON DEVELOPMENT
Edited by Claire B. Kopp

THE CHALLENGE OF CHANGE: PERSPECTIVES ON FAMILY, WORK, AND EDUCATION
Edited by Matina Horner, Carol C. Nadelson, and Malkah T. Notman

THE WOMAN PATIENT
Volume 1: Sexual and Reproductive Aspects of Women's Health Care
Edited by Malkah T. Notman and Carol C. Nadelson

Volume 2: Concepts of Femininity and the Life Cycle
Edited by Carol C. Nadelson and Malkah T. Notman

Volume 3: Aggression, Adaptations, and Psychotherapy
Edited by Malkah T. Notman and Carol C. Nadelson

WOMEN IN MIDLIFE
Edited by Grace Baruch and Jeanne Brooks-Gunn

WOMEN'S PROGRESS: PROMISES AND PROBLEMS
Edited by Jeanne Spurlock and Carolyn B. Robinowitz

WOMEN'S SEXUAL DEVELOPMENT: EXPLORATIONS OF INNER SPACE
Edited by Martha Kirkpatrick

WOMEN'S SEXUAL EXPERIENCE: EXPLORATIONS OF THE DARK CONTINENT
Edited by Martha Kirkpatrick

WOMEN'S PROGRESS
Promises and Problems

Edited by

JEANNE SPURLOCK AND
CAROLYN B. ROBINOWITZ

American Psychiatric Association
Washington, D.C.

PLENUM PRESS • NEW YORK AND LONDON

Library of Congress Cataloging-in-Publication Data

Women's progress : promises and problems / edited by Jeanne Spurlock
  and Carolyn B. Robinowitz.
        p.   cm. -- (Women in context)
    Includes bibliographical references.
    ISBN 0-306-43422-9
    1. Women.   2. Mothers.   3. Family.   I. Spurlock, Jeanne.
  II. Robinowitz, Carolyn.   III. Series.
  HQ1154.W934   1990
  305.4--dc20   90-7175
                                                                   CIP

© 1990 Plenum Press, New York
A Division of Plenum Publishing Corporation
233 Spring Street, New York, N.Y. 10013

Printed in the United States of America

Contributors

Evelia V.-R. Adams • 1207 Summit Avenue, Louisville, Kentucky 40204

Paul L. Adams, M.D. • Private practice, 1169 Eastern Parkway, G–45, Louisville, Kentucky, 40127

Mary S. Akerley, J.D. • Sasscer, Clagett, Channing & Bucher, Upper Marlboro, Maryland 20772

Leona L. Bachrach, Ph.D. • Maryland Psychiatric Research Center, University of Maryland School of Medicine, Cantonsville, Maryland 21228

Elissa P. Benedek, M.D. • Center for Forensic Psychiatry, Ann Arbor, Michigan 48106

Norman R. Bernstein, M.D. • Department of Psychiatry, Harvard Medical School, Cambridge, Massachusetts 02140

Leah J. Dickstein, M.D. • University of Louisville School of Medicine, Louisville, Kentucky 40204

Peggy Dulany • The Synergos Institute, New York, New York 10028

Paul M. Fine, M.D. • Creighton-Nebraska Universities Department of Psychiatry, Omaha, Nebraska 68108

Ruth L. Fuller, M.D. • Department of Psychiatry, University of Colorado Health Sciences Center, School of Medicine, Denver, Colorado 80262

Janice Hutchinson, M.D. • District of Columbia Department of Mental Health, Washington, D.C. 20009

S. Peter Kim, M.D. • Medical College of Georgia, Augusta, Georgia 30912

Martha J. Kirkpatrick, M.D. • Department of Psychiatry, University of California School of Medicine, Los Angeles, California 90024

Mary Pape, M.S. • Iowa Western Community College, Council Bluffs, Iowa 51502

Carolyn B. Robinowitz, M.D. • Office of the Medical Director, American Psychiatric Association, Washington, D.C. 20005

Louise Rogoff-Thompson, Ph.D. • Suburban Mental Health Associates, Baltimore, Maryland 21228

Jeanne Spurlock, M.D. • Office of Minority/National Affairs, American Psychiatric Association, Washington, D.C. 20005

James W. Thompson, M.D., M.P.H. • Department of Psychiatry, University of Maryland School of Medicine, Baltimore, Maryland 21201

Thomas G. Webster, M.D. • George Washington University Medical Center, Washington, D.C. 20037

Virginia N. Wilking, M.D. • Columbia University College of Physicians and Surgeons, New York, New York 10032

Foreword

Now, 25 years into our country's most recent "women's movement" for equality, it is appropriate to reexamine the social and cultural experiences of women. Thanks to the media, researchers, clinicians, and the general public, all are aware that women have been unable to realize many of their goals. At times, distress rather than satisfaction and rejection and disappointment rather than contentment have been the result of the ongoing struggle of women to achieve change—the change in attitudes, behavior, and values necessary to broaden the personal choices and work options open to women.

Nationally recognized authorities on several of the sociocultural issues addressed in this volume, the editors invited noted scholars and clinicians to study some of those issues particularly relevant to women. These include frequently neglected topics, such as the multiplicity of responsibilities of single women and the spectrum of mothering roles, and those more commonly discussed, such as the various roles and patterns in the family, work options and burdens, and interpersonal relationships. The volume provides insightful detail on two prominent and poignant problems of the 1980s—the causes and repercussions of homelessness and sexual life-styles. Such material may facilitate understanding and serve as a catalyst for positive action.

The editors suggest that their volume serve as a model to encourage researchers interested in the issues of women—and men—to investigate other areas of women's lives, areas rife with problems but largely denied or ignored. A paucity of acknowledgment and understanding of the need for change persists in a number of segments of women's life experiences—for example, coping in the later stages of life and with the stresses of a dual career.

The feminist movement of the 19th century had as its goal the right to vote. Our recent women's movement, initiated in the early 1960s and ongoing, seeks broader changes in women's lives and, consequently, in the lives of men. The past two decades of effort have generated personal and cultural turmoil—and change. The changes have been accompanied by an increased awareness of the conflicts felt by some women and the fulfillment of promises experienced by others. I congratulate the editors of this volume and their contributors for highlighting many of the pertinent issues that must be addressed if women—as well as their children and men—are to enjoy the option of a better quality of life.

LEAH J. DICKSTEIN

Louisville, Kentucky

Preface

The idea for this volume grew out of the editors' awareness and concerns that some of the gains of the most recent women's movement were more mythical than real. Although we were convinced that there are greater opportunities and options for women in our society, and particularly for those interested in and committed to pursuing a career, barriers and inequities continue. We recognized, too, the various societal pressures that have an impact on the different life-styles that women have chosen or have had forced upon them. It was upon these reflections that we based the purpose of this volume—to explore current life situations of women and their options for change and growth.

Like the others in the series *Women in Context: Development and Stresses*, this volume is directed to clinicians as well as academicians, including behavioral scientists, educators, nurses, physicians, and social workers. It may be of particular use in women's studies programs.

In developing this volume we sought input from colleagues from various disciplines and asked them to address specific issues from either their personal or professional frame of reference. We are deeply indebted to each of the contributors and thank them for their patience and willingness to respond to what must have seemed to be a myriad of editorial critiques. We are especially appreciative of the editorial services of Joan O'Connor and Elyse Zuckerman, and for the secretarial assistance provided by Hope Ball, Linda Roll, Rosely Stanich, and Lillian Wilson.

JEANNE SPURLOCK, M.D.
CAROLYN B. ROBINOWITZ, M.D.

Contents

Introduction

Jeanne Spurlock and Carolyn B. Robinowitz

A number of events that have taken place during several periods of American history—the 19th-century women's movement, suffrage, social feminism, the Progressive Movement, the women's movement of the 1960s—have heightened women's expectations about choices. Such expectations have led us to believe that we can study for and be successful in those professions and vocations that have been labeled "for men only," or that we could be comfortable about focusing our time and attention on homemaking and childrearing, or that we could do both. We had options! But we also met with barriers. Sometimes these barriers were external to ourselves (e.g., discrimination against women in education and the workplace); in other instances, they may be rooted in our individual makeups.

Our history is replete with examples of the pendulumlike swing of available choices, myths of choices for women subsequent to major social movements. Frequently, women were the "movers" and "shakers" behind the swing toward the maintenance of women's traditional role. For example, a number of local antisuffrage groups, headed by women, united in 1911 to establish the National Association Opposed to the Further Extension of Suffrage to Women (Banner, 1974). The breakup of the family was a powerful antisuffrage argument then, as it is now for the anti-ERA activists.

The identified gains of women's emancipation have sometimes masked the nonchanges and the continued discrimination against women. Banner (1974) made note of this pattern in the 1920s, stating that

> with the exception of their movement into clerical work, women did not substantially improve their position in the labor force in the 1920s. Although

Jeanne Spurlock • Office of Minority/National Affairs, American Psychiatric Association, Washington, D.C. 20005.   Carolyn B. Robinowitz • Office of the Medical Director, American Psychiatric Association, Washington, D.C. 20005.

> the number of women increased in most professions, women still held jobs
> that were less prestigious and lower-paid than those of men (p. 155).

Similar observations have been made in the here and now. The new opportunities have allowed women to be trained for an additional number of "traditionally male" occupations and professions. Yet there remains a wide gender gap in earnings. Our reference to this "down side" is not to discount the fact that women have made it to the near-top in earnings, but to emphasize that the numbers are small, indeed.

Certainly, the pursuit of new opportunities has been a mixed bag for many women. Employment outside the home (which many women must do in order to provide a needed supplement to the family income, or because they are the sole support of the family) has not relieved women of responsibilities of child care and housework. Furthermore, the workplace of new opportunities is often detrimental to the worker's health.

> In addition to older office health problems caused by excessive sitting or standing, fluorescent lighting and ozone from copying machines, clerical workers are exposed to new hazards from computers and office design. . . . "Closed" office buildings, where windows do not open and central air conditioning systems which recirculate filtered air, are leading to a variety of health problems (Gatlin, 1987, p. 228).

The contributors to this volume were invited to address a broad range of societal changes and social issues that have contributed to a wider range of choices for women, as well as issues that have contributed to lessening of options or a second reading of options as myths.

Adams and Adams, in the introductory chapter, recognize the various family structures but give emphasis to a woman and her child (children) as the fundamental family unit. (The editors offer a different opinion in a note at the end of Chapter 1). Illustrations are provided to support their premise that definitions of a family reflect the value of the definer and the particular historical period in which the defining is being done. The authors note also the various political ramifications of family life and functioning.

Spurlock discusses the various assets and liabilities of singleness. Reference is made to the myths that depict single women as unhappy and depressed "rejects" as well as the "other side of the coin" in reporting the views and experiences of never-married women who are voluntarily single and live a full and interesting life.

Fine and Pape focus on foster families and address the myriad problems and joys experienced by foster mothers. Since the majority of children placed in foster care are in trouble, troublesome, and/or severely handicapped, and because placement is designed to be temporary, foster parents are confronted with weighty demands and expectations. The authors call attention to the relatively new trend of ongoing involvement of the birth family in the therapeutic process and, if appropriate, the reunification. As happens in other families, foster mothers usually assume the leading parenting role in these families. Foster parenting is often a family affair, in which birth children and grandparents play a vital role. Fine and Pape point out that the motivations for foster parenting are as varied as those for conceiving and parenting a biological child, or for adoption. The reasons may not be in the best interest of the child. However, unlike birth parents, foster parents are subject to screening. Clinical vignettes are presented to illustrate each of these points. The authors conclude with a list of a variety of resource material for that segment of our readership that is especially interested in foster parenting.

Rogoff-Thompson and Thompson address the various changes that have taken place in the arenas of adoption in recent years: single and older adopting parents, increase in older, handicapped, and mixed-race children. The psychological context of adoption is discussed in terms of losses, particularly as related to the adopting parents, and the multiple ripple effects. Loss by infertility, an experience personally familiar to the authors, is used as a paradigm. Both the birth mother, who gives up her child, and the adopting mother, who is likely to have suffered a loss because of infertility or miscarriage or stillbirth, must work through the grieving and begin to heal before they can find new sources of self-esteem and reintegrate the positive pieces into their respective identities.

Kim also makes note of the changes that have taken place in patterns of adoption over the years, as well as the continuing fluctuations. His focus is identified in his title, "Adopting Children from Other Cultures." He calls attention to the numerous controversies that have been stirred up over transcultural and transracial adoptions, and discusses the problems of cultural dissonance and/or shock. A specific approach for assessment of such problems is presented.

Fuller presents a range of concerns of working mothers—single, married, and divorced—and calls attention to the fact that the numbers of mothers who work outside the home have increased steadily in the past decade. Most experience some guilt about working, regardless of the reason—by choice or because of necessity. Vignettes that describe children's responses to working mothers point up the fallacy of the premise that "latchkey" children, as a whole, are psychologically damaged. However, all working mothers and their children need and benefit from a support network—informal or formal. Fuller highlights reliable child care, which has claimed the attention of government officials as well as employers and parents, as the most important support.

Parenting is likely to be studded with sorrow and pain when a child is developmentally disabled. Akerley and Bernstein address this matter in their respective chapters on the exceptional and mentally retarded children. Ackerley writes as a mother of a child with autism; Bernstein uses his professional experiences as a frame of reference. Both authors underscore the fact that most of the burdens of care fall on the mother, no matter how concerned, enlightened, and supportive the father may be. Chronic stress, constriction of life-styles, and interminable mourning are commonplace. Ackerley's criticism of the helping professions has been heard and responded to by many professionals who have joined parents in forming partnerships in developing and implementing programs for the care of developmentally delayed and mentally ill children.

The content of the section on women with extraordinary problems is likely to be viewed as a strange admixture, especially with the placement of Dulany's piece, "On Becoming Empowered," which stems, in part, from her membership in an influential family. Assets and liabilities have been observed in the life cycle of daughters of widely and well-known figures. Dulany writes about this from the viewpoint of her personal experience. Her contribution to this volume is excerpted from an address that she gave at the Founder's Day celebration at Spelman College in 1983. Dulany's message is applicable to many women, and to all who feel voiceless and ineffective.

A brighter side is extremely dim, if visible at all, for women who abuse their children or for female offenders. Wilking calls our attention to the fact that the actual prevalence of child abuse is not known. Underreporting is suspected, in part because the criteria used to identify abuse vary from state to state. External factors and their internal representations are cited as agents that incite a mother to abuse her child. Considerable psychopathology has been identified in some abusing mothers; deficits in the child might also play a role in the act of abuse. Wilking emphasizes the likelihood of the continuation of abusive patterns in the next generation if early intervention is not accomplished. In view of the long, long history of child abuse, the chances of interrupting the patterns seem bleak unless research findings point to more effective preventive measures and funding is available for the activation of those measures.

Hard data about the prevalence of female crime and delinquency are difficult to locate. Not unlike the reporting of child abuse, many other crimes are not reported. However, the data that are available do *not* lend credence to the premise that there is a link between the emancipation of women and an increase in violent crimes perpetrated by women. As Benedek notes in her introductory statement, violent crimes have been committed by women since the time that Medea murdered to gain her own ends. However, nearly every day we are bombarded with the news of violent crimes carried out by females, including juveniles. Benedek notes that there is relatively little information about recidivism. However, information about the elementary rehabilitation efforts suggest that many, if not most, female offenders have limited options after release from prison.

In her presentation about battered women, Hutchinson points to a number of similarities with female offenders (e.g., the extended history of wife battering, the chronicity of experiences of individual women). Many a battered woman becomes a perpetrator of a violent act when she turns on the batterer after years of victimization. Prevention measures are identified as interventions of choice. The redefining of sex roles was identified as one such measure (e.g., masculinity should not mean the ability to have power or control over another).

Homeless mentally ill women are becoming more visible in large cities across the nation. Bachrach describes them as a very diverse group and emphasizes the changes that have been observed recently—that is, the growing number of younger women and the "new poor." Of equal importance to that of the lack of a home is the absence of affiliative attachments and the prevalence of physical illness among the homeless. The severity and multiplicity of the problems of the homeless mentally ill can accurately be identified as a *crisis* and call for researchers and clinicians to reevaluate their assumptions about this population and the method of intervention. As Bachrach points out, some of the services now provided are not helpful to these individuals who are in life-threatening situations.

Kirkpatrick writes on the growing number of visible one-gender families in the chapter "Homosexuality and Parenting." In keeping with the theme of this volume, Kirkpatrick focuses on lesbian mothers, who appear to be indistinguishable from single heterosexual mothers in childrearing. Not unlike those of the "true" families described by Adams and Adams, the lives of lesbian mothers are organized around their children.

In the final chapter Webster provides pertinent information about the choices, or lack of choices, available to female transsexuals. His accounts of the struggles that these women have with their gender identity are culled from his own clinical experiences, as a member of a team of clinicians and investigators of a gender identity program, and from an extensive review of the literature. Webster reinforces the need for attention to be given to further research as to etiology, and work that will lead to public understanding and interventions that will allow female transsexuals significant options that can be pursued more easily.

We are aware that a number of topics (e.g., elderly women, minority women who are in positions of double/triple jeopardy) have not been dealt with at all or in depth. We welcome and encourage our readers to pick up where we have left off.

REFERENCES

Banner, L. W. (1974). *Women in modern America* (2nd ed.). San Diego: Harcourt Brace.
Gatlin, R. (1987). *American women since 1945*. Jackson: University of Mississippi Press.

PART I

Some Family Structures

Chapter 1

What Is a Woman's Family? Fluctuations in Definitions, Structure, and Functions

Evelia V.-R. Adams and Paul L. Adams

A family can be a group of 20 or more persons; it can include only 2. It can be an elaborate reticulum of "invisible loyalties" that extend across decades, generations, and centuries to give a person a sense of family identity and feelings of pride; it may last but a few days. Or it may begin but never be completed in the sense of having two parents living with the child(ren). A family usually is a small group of people living face-to-face and *tête-à-tête*, forming intense affiliations and conflicts, loving and hating in highly charged situations.

DEFINITION

Families are relatively small. A very large family is still a rather small group in urban America. Since families are units that census takers find it difficult to manage, the social statistics in the United States generally are based on households, not on families. When a household has a true family within it, it still is smaller in size than, for example, a young adults' commune or a regathering of elderly brothers and sisters with their spouses. The American family now has an average of between one and two children, culminating a decline in average family size that commenced in the 17th century. Historian Carl N. Degler (1980) sees the decline in fertility rates (7.04 children on the average in 1800, 3.56 on the average in 1900, and 1.9 on the average in 1980) as the most important

Evelia V.-R. Adams • 1207 Summit Avenue, Louisville, Kentucky 40204.   Paul L. Adams • Private practice, 1169 Eastern Parkway, G–45, Louisville, Kentucky 40127.

datum about women in families in America. In the United States, families get smaller each decade both because more adults flee from them and because fewer children are born into them.

The sociologist Helena Z. Lopata (1973) advanced an overly literal and concrete definition when she toyed with the question: What is a family? "The basic family, then, consists of people united through marriage or birth, who share a common household and carry out activities which make living together possible" (Lopata, 1973, p. 1).

Quickly thereafter, attentive to numerous exceptions to her own definition of a family, Lopata nodded toward some contemporary experimentation and concluded that the actual family situation is "very revolutionary."

> Communal living . . . [h]omosexual unions, delayed marriage, adoption of children in the absence of either mother or father, the refusal to add to the population explosion by having children, the serious occupational or career involvement of wives, career shifts by middle-aged husbands, foster grandparenthood, cohabitation of the elderly who are unwilling to lose the benefits of pensions and Social Security through marriage, same-age communities isolated from the problems of the other generations, leisure focus rather than work motivation—all these experiments indicate a decision by some people to break with the past in terms of heterosexual family roles. (Lopata, 1973, p. 9)

That Lopata's first definition of the basic family was a conventional one is readily apparent. She underlined the traditional tie-in of family and marriage. Of course, a family is a grouping of people who "share a common household." The group's members do share living space in order to care for their basic needs, and the group's members usually are "united through marriage or birth." The conventional wisdom holds that a marital pair is a kind of precondition of family life. However, this criterion has not endured over the years.

Although a woman living with and caring for a child is *the fundamental family unit*, we are aware that there are many other kinds of *households* that approach family status. In Table 1, we have depicted the many "family types" that might engage a woman. Only Types IA and B and IIA and B, marked with asterisks, are true families by our definition; those groups that lack the two generations are not true families. Such groups and individuals, however, do think of themselves as families. Table 1 does not contain those "families" in which there is no woman, of course, since that is not our current focus.

EYE OF THE BEHOLDER

Whatever a woman's family is, its definition reflects the value of the definer, the spirit of one's era, and one's particular social perspective. A few examples of the different perceptions of a family are reviewed.

Table 1. Women in Families[a]

I.   Types of family participated in by developing females
*A.   Family of one's childhood: family of orientation
*B.   Family of one's motherhood: family of procreation
C.   Family of one's senescence: "family" of empty nest (conjugal pair or alone)
II. Types of household forms involving women
*A.   "Complete" families with plural generations and adults of both genders
1. Nuclear, with child focus
2. Nuclear, with conjugal focus
3. Extended, with or without joint residence
4. Communal
*B.   "Partial" families with children in female-headed households
1. Formerly complete, now eroded or broken
a. By death
b. By divorce
c. By legal separation
d. By desertion
e. By father's work-related absence
2. Never completed or never fathered
a. By out-of-wedlock parentage
b. By breaking up conjugal pair during pregnancy
3. One-gender couples living with children
4. One-gender trios or communes with children
C.   "Families" of adults only (pairs, trios, etc.)
1. Two genders (e.g., both sexes but childless)
2. One gender (e.g., homosexual or other pairs of women)
3. Communal (e.g., convents, women's communes, co-ops, or dormitories)
D.   One-person households (a woman alone)

[a]Families marked with asterisks are discussed in the text.

For the economist, the family is an arrangement for transferring income from workers and producers to nonproducing consumers, from productive individuals to those who are helpless, dependent, enfeebled, or handicapped. Primary among the world's helpless consumers are young children, a realistic economic burden to working parents everywhere.

For someone who defines the family in a religious mode, the family is an arrangement both temporal and eternal whereby mating, procreating, birth, growth, and dying all are imbued with a transcendent meaning, aligning individuals and groups into more harmonious relations with one another and even with impersonal, higher powers.

From a biologic perspective, a family is an instrument for controlled reproduction, replenishment (whether degrading or uplifting) of the species, begetting and nurturing of children, so that *they* may have their turn—grow to puberty and maturity, mate, replenish the species, and nourish a succeeding generation.

For an educator or behavior modifier, the family is a training field *par excellence*, unmatched for its power to condition the young. Educationally speaking, it can be said that the family retains a paraphrase of the motto ascribed to the Roman Catholic Church, "Give me a child till she is seven and she will be mine for the rest of her life." The strength of early childhood learning surpasses that of all later life. Indeed, the family gets there early and in force, engendering a child's basic attitudes about her body, gender, and self by the time she is 3 years old, not 7 (Adams-Tucker & Adams, 1980).

An expert in politics sees the family as itself a political unit, a microcosm of the larger *polis*, and a prestage for the individual's citizenship. As the family tests and "checks out" the child's capabilities for bonding or attachment, for dependency, self-assertion, submission, defiance, initiative, industry, mastery, and aggression, some profound political shapings occur. Uttering more truth than poetry, Bernard de Mandeville (cited in Adams, Berg, Berger, Duane, Neill, & Ollendorff, 1971) wrote:

"It is our Parents, that first cure us of natural Wildness, and break in us the Spirit of Independency we are all born with: It is to them that we owe the first Rudiments of our Submission; and to the Honour and Deference which Children pay to Parents, all societies are obliged for the Principle of Human Obedience." Today's family has a guaranteed primacy in the life of either the person or the milieu only when the community is small and relatively isolated. When the size of the community enlarges, or as it increases its interpenetration with other communities, or as urbanism replaces agrarianism, the influence of the family lessens for its members and for the community at large.

Because life expectancy has advanced upward, both one's first family and one's family of procreation today take up a proportionally smaller segment of the life-span than in earlier epochs. When women died at 40 years of age, they spent roughly half their lives with father and mother and the other half with husband and offspring. Today, the fractions are assorted differently, since many women postpone childbearing until near the end of their reproductive years, and others, at an earlier age, limit the number of children they bear; others choose not to bear children. Often, one-fourth of a woman's life-span is spent in her family of orientation, perhaps another one-fourth or one-third in her family of procreation, and then three-eighths to one-half of her days are spent in an "empty nest," often in prolonged widowhood for many of her latest years.

For some, a "family" is any cohabiting couple, group, or commune who provide that person with "a haven in a heartless world." For others, the family is oppression and bondage from which one seeks only liberation. For many individuals, especially the working class, the family is the central focus of all life and the gauge for measuring all of one's endeavors and gains. For the upper middle class, the family is purely individualistic and expressive, a spontaneity theater in which each character learns how to act, think, and feel for purposes of self-expression or fuller self-development. The family is a single membrane of undifferentiated egos; the family is a system organized to collectivize and then to hatch out individuals with all their special *individuality*. The family breeds both sociability and uniqueness.

CASE. An adopted child named Melinda, a girl of 11 years, had some very definite views about the family. Her biologic mother and father had grown up in underorganized yet complete nuclear families. Both had been poor from birth onward, and after their marriage in their midteens, they grossly neglected their firstborn daughter, Melinda. That was "Family 1" for her. When the child was 2½ years old, the parents battered her and scalded her badly. Skin grafts were required. The welfare department began a long haul of trying to support and trust Melinda's parents. Ultimately, the welfare department gained custody. After recurrent abuse, parental rights were terminated legally when Melinda was 5 years old.

Melinda was adopted from ages 5½ to 8½ by a middle-class couple. When the adoptive parents divorced, they no longer wanted Melinda and gave custody back to the welfare department, thereby ending Melinda's "Family 2" through "de-adoption."

From ages 8½ to 11, Melinda lived in a series of foster and group homes over a wide area of two different states. At age 11, she was adopted by a childless divorcee, and she settled into her third "real family" in time to stabilize for a puberty and adolescence that gave promise of being rocky at best. A child such as Melinda idealizes and reveres "The Family" but might acknowledge that only her third family, with a single parent, showed prospects of meeting her needs as a young person.

COMMENT. By her 11th year, Melinda had had a gruesome family experience with those who "begat" her, a great disappointment when her adoptive parents obtained an annulment of the adoption when they divorced, and several unhappy fostering experiences. Ultimately, she found herself in a two-person, two-generation, one-gender adoptive family that promised something positive for Melinda's life. The comments of children like Melinda about family life might be less prosaic and more realistic than those of the behavioral scientists.

FUNCTIONS OF A FAMILY FOR ADULTS, CHILDREN, AND SOCIETY

The family, in truth, has both individual and societal functions. We acknowledge that the needs of adults and children differ, and that their needs are met (or not met) differently within ordinary families. Consequently, we find it prudent to divide the family's individual functions according to those for adults and those for a child and then briefly discuss what a family is good for—its societal functions.

For an adult person, the functions of a procreative family with two parents are at least four: (a) psychic security derived from companionship and interdependence, (b) psychic security derived from parenting, (c) sexual gratification with a relatively durable partner, and (d) physical security from being in an economic unit that will attend to one's needs and wants "in sickness and in health." It must be noted that the identified functions, except parenting, pertain to childless couples as well.

Of all the social institutions and arrangements, the family is most intimately incorporative of individuals. The family is nearly inescapable once it has formed. An adult may exert political or economic or other forms of influence by designating proxies and representatives, but in the family it is more likely one's bodily presence that is demanded and really counts. In the family, one's role depends on one's being there; substitutes for oneself are awkward even when they try to stand in only briefly. The family is not like an ordinary work group in which roles and tasks can be shifted around, covered by others, delegated and reshuffled with little trouble. In the family the unique person is what matters, so the family has untold import as a life-organizer for the adult person. Wifing and mothering can give a woman a place in her scheme of things that she could not obtain elsewhere. Securities and comforts abound in a family that functions well; troubles are rampant when functioning becomes impaired.

Yet the family apparently is optional behavior for adults; they can remain unmarried if they wish and barren if they choose. Almost no one is forced to form a family of procreation, but most people choose to do so. The social patterning that leads us to that choice is imperious and totalitarian, perhaps, for being informal. It is a conditioning of our hopes and behavior, which is based on no laws that make family building compulsory. And there are no specified penalties levied for not forming a family. Instead, the "reproduction of mothering" (Chodorow, 1978) turns out to have roots in early childhood, based on the ways the mother treated her daughter, molded her, and taught her to feel about her femaleness and femininity. It is nearly a matter of imprinting mothering on the little girl during her infancy. For such a woman, everything feels right (at least a good part of the time) as she engages in making a family when she becomes an adult.

For a child, her family of orientation is her instrumentality for life itself by furnishing (a) physical security as a consumer and (b) psychic security or ego identity. Being helpless and dependent, a child needs to consume loving care in order to survive. A child is only a consumer of goods and services for the first 3 or 7 years of life, after which age, in much of human history, children have begun to contribute to, not just to take from, the adults within the family.

In the United States, childhood ends and, *pari passu*, the young adult starts producing and taking certain liberties at variable ages that depend on specific behaviors. For example, in some states of the United States, a woman may consent to nonmarital intercourse only at 18 years, may drive a car at 16, may marry at 14, may not buy whiskey before age 21. The school-leaving age ordinarily is 16 years, and that is when most working-class people ascribe childhood's termination as occurring. In some families, childhood ends earlier; in others, later.

Some psychiatrists and other behavioral scientists see puberty as the end of "latency" or middle childhood and as the onset of *adolescence.* Thereby, they insert adolescence as an interstage of human development, a socially ordained delay or moratorium before childhood's irresponsibility must be given up. But both childhood and adolescence generally are lived out within the confines of the family.

For the society, a family of two parents and one or more children subserves several vital functions:

1. Procreation: Most children are born into a complete family and spend important parts of their lives in a complete family. Hence, the family traditionally functions as society's seedbed.

2. Education: Even a one-parent family serves as a unit for the socialization of children, the channeling and patterning of child behavior into conformity to the norms of society as a whole.

3. Regulation of sexuality: Marital behavior and the sexual norms of society are upheld to the extent that adults confine their major expressions of sexual intercourse to the marriage relationship. Most societies (a) favor marital (more than premarital or extramarital) sexuality, (b) outlaw incest and adultery, and (c) set up certain sanctions to discourage—while providing some exceptions—sexuality, such as fornication or mismating.

4. Home economics: At times in U.S. history, a woman's family has been the basic economic unit for the society. Within its context, there have been produced, distributed, and consumed the core economic goods of food, shelter, clothing, and the implements for farming and hunting. Today, although cottage industries are relatively rare, the family unit persists as the fundamental arena for income transfer in every society. The family sees to it that the wages of producers, as well as the state's family supplements and bonuses, are transferred into the hands and mouths of the dependent members of society, the nonproductive consumers who are too elderly, infirm, or young to work and earn

wages themselves. In the United States, a major yet inadequate welfare program is Aid to Families with Dependent Children (AFDC).

5. Health delivery: Most of the world's health maintenance is carried out within the family. Moreover, most of the prevention of disability and disorder, including mental illnesses, is done within the family group. Workers "stay home" when they are ill; it is at home that most nursing care is administered by family members. Sometimes, too, kinship gives a weak counteraction to sickness (Parsons & Fox, 1952).

6. Social order and control: When family members can be made docile, that is done within the family. When adults or children cannot be brought to conform within the family, they usually are just as incorrigible outside the family; if the family cannot do it, hardly any other instrumentality can. Particularly for adults, the family is a prime example of their predictable and reliable behavior, and that, after all, is what constitutes any institution. The family is society's basic institutional ground.

It is worth a special notation at this point that a mother-only family household, a one-parent family headed by a woman, can make rather good approximations of all the functions listed *as long as it is not poverty-stricken* (Adams, Milner, & Schrepf, 1984). The only things missing are the companionship and regulated heterosexuality of a complete family, although the income to be transferred usually is reduced greatly.

More Than Three

It is said frequently that a woman lives in three families in the course of a life (see Table 1). She lives first in her baby family or family of origin. More aptly, we believe, it should be called her *family of orientation*, for it is the small group in which she first gets her bearings on what it is to be human and interdependent, on what it is to receive nurture and gratification, on what her body feels like to her and how to image her body, and on what it is to be female and to feel more or less good in one's own self-esteem. Second, having had her personhood oriented in her first family, she helps to form her *family of procreation*, the family in which she is at the helm at least as copilot and perhaps the only head of her household containing children. Third, a woman may form a "reconjugalized" family with the same man or with another person when her children will have grown up, leaving a residual, *empty nest family*. Each of those three types has a very different aura—and meaning—for the woman.

We believe that most women have many more families and homes than the three cited. Each home and family carries its own style, flavor, ambiance, and spirit. Some of the multiple varieties of family living are illustrated by the lives of the two authors of this chapter. For the sake of emphasis on the female, we shall focus on the families experienced by Evelia (EV-RA). These are laid out succinctly in Table 2, showing some geographic mobility, variegated compositions of households, and innumerable stresses at different developmental steps in the family experiences of one woman.

Table 2. Household Composition for EV-RA at Various Periods[a]

*Family 1	Mother, Father, EV-RA, and paternal grandmother, two unmarried paternal uncles, paternal aunt, and her husband—in Havana, Cuba
Family 2	Same as 1, but *sister* added
Family 3	Same as 2, but paternal uncle 1 left home
Family 4	Same as 3, but paternal uncle 2 left home
Family 5	Same as 4, but paternal aunt's divorced husband left the household
*Family 6	Paternal aunt and paternal grandmother left the home; *mother, father, EV-RA, and her sister* remaining
Family 7	Paternal family house sold, and Family 6 now moved to maternal grandmother's home; family now consists of *mother, father, EV-RA* (age 4 years), *sister* and maternal grandmother, three maternal aunts (1, 3, 4), and two maternal uncles
Family 8	Same as 7, except maternal aunt 2 married and left the home
Family 9	Same as 8, except maternal uncle 2 sent to manage family farm 80 miles away
Family 10	Same as 9, except maternal aunt 3 married and moved out to live with her husband's extended family
Family 11	Same as 10, except maternal uncle 2 married and moved
Family 12	Same as 11, except maternal aunt 2 (divorced) and her daughter came to live in household
Family 13	Maternal uncle 2 returned to the home with his wife
Family 14	Maternal aunt 2 and daughter departed when aunt 2 remarried
Family 15	*Father* left for 6 months to visit USSR, returned to spend 6 months as political prisoner
Family 16	*Father* and *mother* divorced; father left the home
Family 17	Maternal uncle 2 divorced wife, and she left; *mother, EV-RA, sister*, and maternal grandmother, maternal uncle 2, maternal aunt 4 remained
Family 18	Maternal uncle 2 remarried, left to live in new wife's extended family's home
Family 19	Maternal grandmother died
Family 20	*Mother* remarried and her new husband joined the household
Family 21	*Sister* married, moved out
Family 22	*EV-RA* emigrated and shared an apartment with two young women
*Family 23	*EV-RA* married *PLA* who had *daughter* by previous marriage
*Family 24	*Daughter* born; family of procreation now established
Family 25	*EV-RA, PLA, stepdaughter*, and *daughter* lived 2 months with mother-in-law in a second city
Family 26	Same as 25, except for mother-in-law, in a third city
Family 27	Same as 26, plus *son* born; family of procreation living in a fourth city
Family 28	Same as 27, with *EV-RA's* sister and her son, refugees, now joining household in a fifth city

(continued)

Table 2. (Continued)

Family 29	Same as 28, with elderly German refugee friend added to the household
Family 30	Same as 28, when friend left
Family 31	Same as 27, when *sister* and her son left
Family 32	Same as 31, except *stepdaughter* left for college
Family 33	Same as 31, when *stepdaughter* returned from college
Family 34	Same as 31, except *stepdaughter* moved out and subsequently married
Family 35	*EV-RA's mother*, suffering from amyotrophic lateral sclerosis, joined family
Family 36	Same as 32, when *mother* returned to her homeland to die
Family 37	*Daughter* moved out to commune
Family 38	*EV-RA, PLA, and son* moved to a sixth city
Family 39	*Son* went to boarding school
Family 40	*Son* back from school, home now in a seventh city
Family 41	*Son* moved in and out, with several companions
*Family 42	*EV-RA and PLA*; "empty nest" family of senescence

*a*Families (households) marked with asterisks are discussed in the text.

EV-RA's 42 different households were, in reality, more diverse than depicted in Table 2: Live-in household servants changed, mainly reduced by attrition from five to two in number. In a profound sense, those employees were integral members of the families, which they both served and bossed (numbers 1 through 21 in Table 2). Part-time employees of the household—a laundress, a governess and tutor, a seamstress—also influenced the coloration of the extended, multigenerational family during shorter blocks of time. Also, since EV-RA married, the family of procreation was augmented, in a style more North American than Cuban, by numerous friends (not relatives) who lived with the family for periods of less than 6 months. Hence, an accurate listing would show many more types of households than those charted.

It is small wonder, considering the mobility of persons and families and the fact that families move through cycles of buildup, integration, hatching, and dispersion, that one person can experience over a period of slightly more than 50 years so intricate and diverse an array of families. EV-RA lived mainly in two grandparental *extended* households, while the grandparents' offspring were maturing and departing, then in a *nuclear family of orientation*, then in a *nuclear family of procreation*, and currently in the family of her growing old, a *conjugal* family of two persons, physically living together but spiritually inclusive of a multitude of invisible although significant others. Thus, it is that an "empty nest" does not mean an empty life or a loss of dynamic relationships.

Evelia's Family 1 was based on her paternal grandmother's nuclear family as it became an extended family. Into the ranks of her widowed paternal grandmother, two parental uncles, and an aunt, Evelia's mother and father were the first conjugal pair to be brought into the extended family. When Evelia (and her only sister) were born, a completed nuclear family was present, nuclear but enfolded in an extended family of the father's kinfolk.

Family 6 showed, as the remnant of Evelia's much pruned-down first extended family, a nuclear bigenerational family purely and simply: two parents and their daughters—but not for long. Family 1 through 21 showed Evelia living in another extended family—with numerous changes—based on the cohabitation and dispersion of her mother's kinfolk. Cuba in those days favored the sustenance of nuclear families within the bosom of larger kin groups.

Family 23 was something new under the sun for Evelia. By marrying, she entered a denuded family of father and daughter, thereby reconstituting a stepfamily, and, after a daughter was born, a completed nuclear family of procreation—Family 24, a nuclear group augmented with the birth of her son and final child as Family 27.

Kellam (1977) at the University of Chicago has described 86 types of households (according to the component members) in Woodlawn, a black ghetto area of Chicago. Family diversity in all economic classes is an unquestionable reality today. The structures, functions, and operating processes of "normal" or well-functioning families have been described from many vital perspectives in a good resource book, *Normal Family Processes* (Walsh, 1982).

SUMMARY AND CONCLUSIONS

Having defined the family as a bigenerational group living together in intimate face-to-face relationships, we advanced the viewpoint that the most truncated actual woman's family that we can conceive of is a mother-and-child dyad. All "true" families contain that basic nucleus if they contain a grown woman. And, if there is no adult female to play the caretaking role, a family must have a grown male who carries out child caretaking functions in lieu of a mothering person. According to our definition, there can be no family if there are no children present. We see other units as approximations of a family, as households only. Women assuredly live in a plethora of such childless households in the 1980s.

Families may exist whenever an adult male and/or an adult female *and children* cohabit and interact. Complete families may have a child focus or an adult focus; they may be nuclear or extended groupings, and they may be communal, at least in some of the current experimentations that we have observed. Families do exist whenever a single parent lives with a child or children; the parent may be a mother or a father *or a surrogate of either one.* When children are *born into* a one-parent family, as occurs with over half of black infants born in the United States, they frequently have been said to be illegitimate, a labeling that serves to shift blame or stigma onto such children, not their parents.

When children are born into completed families that subsequently become eroded or broken, to be headed by the mother, such children often are more respectable but equally neglected by the society around them. One-parent families (especially the more numerous ones that are headed by women) are families at risk economically, politically, and from the standpoint of esteem and honor, but in spite of everything, they do persist and multiply.

Scattered but seriously conducted studies suggest that one-gender couples living with children may build an effective family, too, seen from the vantage point of the children. The same would seem to be even more true of one-gender trios or larger groups living communally. There are numerous interesting innovations showing great variation on the basic nurturant adult and child family.

Women derive considerable satisfaction and security when, at different times in the life cycle, they may live in quasi-families—e.g., with a member of the opposite or same sex but without children. Women derive considerable satisfaction from communal living arrangements. Many women who live in quasi-families or live alone have contributed significantly to the well-being of members of family units, which we have identified as true families. This certainly has been our experience.

At the risk of overstating the case, we have chosen to emphasize not sameness but difference, differentness, and fluidity in family composition and functioning. The family spectrum is here to stay, and to continue involving women very profoundly, so long as nurturance of young human persons remains a positive value—for even a minority, in an otherwise antichild, antiwoman, and antiwelfare nation. All families are jeopardized in such a nation, and children as a class are imperiled and at risk.

What does the future hold for the family spectrum, for the "intact, nuclear family"? As Engels (1902) wrote of future socialist generations, which he envisioned would follow him, we, too, suspect that, with or without a socialist economy, "they will not give a moment's thought to what we today believe should be their course. They will follow their own practice and fashion their own public opinion. . ." (p. 100).

Editors' Note. The editors take strong exception to the authors' definitions of "true" and "quasi" families. We have known many childless families and single adults who are integral members of a family. As noted in a task force report of the American Psychiatric Association (1986), "Living alone does not imply the absence of family membership or family ties" (p. 19). Furthermore, the report noted that "the term 'family,' like 'music,' almost defies definition. Everyone knows what it is, but hardly anyone can say what it is. Individual experience and preference vary tremendously" (p. 1).

In his analysis of Afro-American families as a social system, Billingsley (1968) describes some family units as without children. The "incipient, extended, augmented family," consisting of a marital couple, other relatives, and nonrelatives, is illustrative. Nonrelatives as members of a family also are discussed by Stack (1974).

This difference of opinion is not stated to diminish the importance of families that bear and rear children but to identify these families as one of several types. We concur with the authors' view that "whatever a woman's family is, its definition reflects the value of the definer, the spirit of one's era, and one's particular social perspective."

REFERENCES

Adams, P., Berg, L., Berger, N., Duane, M., Neill, A. S., & Ollendorff, R. (1971). *Children's rights*. New York: Praeger.

Adams, P., Milner, J., & Schrepf, N. (1984). *Fatherless children*. New York: Wiley Interscience.

Adams-Tucker, C., & Adams, P. (1980). Role of the father. In M. Kirkpatrick (Ed.), *Women's sexual development*. New York: Plenum.

American Psychiatric Association. (1986). *Changing family patterns in the United States*. Washington, DC: Author.

Billingsley, A. (1968). *Black families in white America*. Englewood Cliffs, NJ: Prentice-Hall.

Chesler, P. (1986). *Mothers on trial*. New York: McGraw-Hill.

Chodorow, N. (1978). *The reproduction of mothering: Psychoanalysis and the sociology of gender*. Berkeley: University of California Press.

Degler, C. N. (1980). *At odds: Women and the family in America from the revolution to the present*. New York: Oxford University Press.

Engels, F. (1902). *The origin of the family, private property, and the state*. Chicago: Kerr.

Kellam, S. G., Ensminger, M. E., & Turner, R. J. (1977). Family structure and the mental health of children. *Archives of General Psychiatry, 34*, 1012–1022.

Lopata, H. (1973). *Marriages and families*. New York: Van Nostrand.

Parsons, T., & Fox, R. (1952). Illness, therapy, and the modern urban American family. *Journal of Social Issues, 13*, 31–44.

Stack, C. B. (1974). *All our kin: Strategies for survival in a black community*. New York: Harper Colophon.

Walsh, F. (Ed.). (1982). *Normal family processes*. New York: Guilford Press.

Chapter 2

Single Women

JEANNE SPURLOCK

> *Single is a word used to categorize a vast and divergent group of persons in order to treat them on the basis of one common criterion—their non marriage. . . . We lack the word to describe persons who lead lives, hold jobs, have fun, experience hard times; in short, who do all things persons do, but who prefer not to be married.*
>
> STEIN, 1976

A number of definitions have been ascribed to singleness: never married, divorced (shortly or long after marriage), or widowed. Traditionally, single women have been identified as never married and usually childless (Adams, 1976). The latter criterion has varied in different subcultures and socioeconomic groups in the United States. Never-married, middle-class, heterosexual, usually childless women who are over 30 years of age will be the subject of this chapter. These women fall into three categories: those who deliberately delay marriage until completion of professional training, those who are voluntarily single (singleness declared as a preferred life-style), and those who are involuntarily single (marriage preferred, but thwarted by various factors). Data were obtained from open-ended interviews* and other contacts (in social and work-related settings) with single women. All of these women had received formal education beyond high school—college or business. Most were college graduates, and a sizable number had graduated from a professional school.

A woman's classification may vary from one period of time to another. Betty, now age 60, was determined to finish postgraduate training in pediatrics and establish an academic-clinical career before marrying. As she approached the mid-30s she was eager to be married, but her

---

*The assistance of Nora D. Vasquez is acknowledged with appreciation.

JEANNE SPURLOCK • Office of Minority/National Affairs, American Psychiatric Association, Washington, D.C. 20005.

choices were dwindling. She turned down a marriage proposal on her 41st birthday: "He just wasn't the right person for me." She became convinced that "marriage for the sake of being married" was not for her. Shortly, thereafter, Betty identified herself as fitting in the group of "voluntary singles."

WHO ARE THE NEVER-MARRIED WOMEN?

Figures presented in Table 1, excerpted from the U.S. Bureau of the Census, Current Population Reports, illustrate the shifts that take place from one period of time to another, and female–male comparisons.

The fact that women, as a group, married at a later age in the 1980s than in the previous decade probably accounts for the increase of single women in the 30 to 34 age bracket in 1985. No hard data were found to explain the reduction of numbers of single women in the 55 to 64 and 65 to 74 age spans and/or the increase (although slight) in the age group of 75 and older.

Single women are from all ethnic and racial groups and religious backgrounds. Some work at low-level, low-paying jobs; others hold high-level executive positions and may or may not be paid at the same level as their male counterparts. Some have taken early retirement. Some have been formally retired for a number of years but are active volunteers in various arenas of service; others are content (or discontent) to pursue an interest that was submerged in previous years. Some single women, at all ages, are in excellent health; others experience a range of health problems. Feminists and traditionalists are represented in the group, as are various personality types. The representation among sin-

Table 1. Single (Never-Married) Persons As Percent of Total Population, by Age and Sex: 1975–1986[a]

	Male				Female			
Age	1975	1980	1985	1986	1975	1980	1985	1986
30–34	11.1	15.9	20.8	22.2	7.5	9.5	13.5	14.2
35–39	8.6	7.8	10.1	11.2	5.0	6.2	8.1	8.4
40–44	7.2	7.1	8.6	8.5	4.8	4.8	5.3	5.5
45–54	6.3		6.1	5.9	4.6	4.7	4.6	4.7
55–64	4.7	4.9	5.3	5.1	5.1	4.5	3.7	3.9
65 and older	4.7	4.9	5.3	5.1	5.8	5.9	5.1	5.2
65–74	4.3	5.2	5.2	5.2	5.8	5.6	4.4	4.4
75 and older	5.5	4.2	5.3	5.0	5.8	6.3	6.2	6.3

[a]Source: U.S. Bureau of the Census, Current Population Reports, series P-20, No. 418, and earlier reports.

gle women in each of the aforementioned categories is no different than in the group of married or previously married women.

NEGATIVE AND POSITIVE IMAGES

Simon (1987) refers to the Anglo-American culture's labeling of unmarried women as "a bundle of negative personal characteristics, and a metaphor for barrenness, ugliness, and death" (p. 2). Furthermore, the author notes that the negativity of singleness has been incorporated into the child's card game of Old Maid. In order to win, players must not be caught with the "old maid" card in their hand.

The undesirability of singleness has been advanced by poets and novelists, as well as behavioral and social scientists. Simon's (1987) illustrations include William Wordsworth's bemoaning "maidens withering on the stalk" and William Faulkner's reference, "He was as crochety about his julep as an old maid, measuring everything by a recipe in his head."

Never-married women have been labeled as second-class citizens, making the best of being without a man. From this premise springs the notion that single women *must* be unhappy and lonely (Hunter College Women's Studies Collective, 1983). Single women have been labeled as shriveled and withered sexually, or, as occurred in the area of sexual liberation of the 1960s, as loose and immoral on the one hand and "with it" on the other.

Adams (1976) suggested that single women are often viewed in negative terms because of the widely held concept that women are not married because of psychological deficits. Women who declare their pleasures and satisfaction in being single have been said to be rationalizing, or that they are utilizing the defense of denial. Staples (1979) adds to the view of single black women as rejects by his statements about black men's disdain of strong women and his conclusion that single black women are given low scores on the femininity scale.

Certainly, the image making does not occur in a vacuum. The events that take place in the environment of the broad political arenas are factors of considerable influence. At one time in American history, a married woman's dependence upon her husband was expected, at least among the white middle class. However, our various wars brought about significant changes in this concept and economic dependency/independency of womenkind. At such times, thoughts about economic security are less likely to be considered as a motivating factor for marriage, and efforts directed toward independence and singleness take on a more positive light. The politics of employment of the 1870s is illustrative. A national teacher shortage, created by the expansion of public education, provided increased opportunities for women teachers. The fact that a single status was one of the few requirements brought some positivity to the image of unmarried women. Since teaching was one of the very few white-collar occupations open to blacks, the changes in the educational system were of particular significance in altering the image of single black women. Woloch (1984) noted that spinsters "moved from the periphery of history to the center stage" (p. 274) in the late 1800s.

> During Jane Addams's life time, single women became the advance troops of New Women, assuming highly visible leadership roles in the professions, reforms, and women's education. Jane Addams was not an isolated example but part of a large cohort of unmarried women leaders, including Lillian Wald in the settlement movement, Frances Willard in the temperance movement, Anna Howard Shaw in the suffrage movement, M. Carey Thomas in women's higher education, and all of the Hull House inner circle. During the progressive era, when women's impact on public life reached a new high, more single women were at the peak of their careers, in proportion to all women, than at any time, before or since.

A number of factors have been cited that account for the increase in single women in that particular era and the advance they made in professional and civic circles. Not the least important were the decline in the number of eligible men, and the increased and improved options that women had for "higher education, professional employment and for establishing supportive relationships with women outside the family" (Woloch, 1984, p. 275). These factors continue to be operative. The need for economic security is no longer a reason for a large percentage of women to seek marriage. In many circles, women are no longer viewed as accessories to men, or as social rejects, if they happen to be single. The use of the title Ms has served to diminish the emphasis that had long been placed on a woman's marital status (Hunter College Women's Studies Collective, 1983). However, a woman's single status continues to be viewed less than positively by many individuals. A male associate confided that when he is in doubt about the marital status of women to whom he is writing business letters, he uses the title Mrs. He has assumed that women would prefer to be misidentified as married rather than as single.

LIVING SINGLE

HOUSING. Housing is less likely to be a problem for single women who are economically secure. Certainly they have more options than single women on low and fixed incomes in urban communities. Safety and discrimination add to the problems generated by high rents. Stein (1976) writes of reports of landlords openly stating their preference for married couples because of their perception that single persons party too much and make for considerable traffic and noise. Single women have been questioned about their ability to pay the rent without outside assistance, the implication being that they were likely to be prostitutes, or that they would default. A single professional woman in her 40s indicated interest in buying a large cooperative apartment that became available when the couple who owned the property was selling because of their impending divorce. She was startled to hear the soon-to-be-divorced woman, who was also a professional person, inquire why a single woman would need or want such a large apartment.

Some single women have solved the problems created by cost and safety by renting an apartment in a suburban community and commuting (by bus or train) to their place of work in the city. Sandra, a 32-year-old government employee, was able to afford an automobile (which allowed for weekend jaunts) because of the savings accumulated as a result of lower costs involved in the purchase of a condominium apartment in the suburbs. Another bonus was the large number of other singles in the complex and the various social outlets that were generated by the residents.

Other never-married women have been successful in finding compatible individuals to share the cost of renting a large enough house or apartment to afford privacy for each individual. Such arrangements have been made successfully in cities as well as in the suburban communities. Single women who are well off financially have selected a single-family dwelling in the city or nearby suburban community; others choose an apartment or townhouse in a neighborhood of their choice.

Housing arrangements vary from one period in the life cycle to another. At age 55, Frances chose to move to a larger apartment in order to bring her aging mother to live with her and to provide accommodations for a practical nurse, when/if such assistance might be needed. Her mother, a woman of independent means and character, was very much involved in the making of this decision, a move that worked out well since both have been able to maintain considerable privacy. This arrangement would probably not have gone so smoothly if this mother and daughter had not also been good friends.

Some single women choose to move to a retirement community as they approach old age. In such communities, one is able to live alone and, at the same time, have immediate access to any emergency service that might be needed. In her survey of single women, Simon (1987) reported that

> with few exceptions, the never married women . . . viewed old age as a time in which to pool resources and share living quarters with a friend or sibling. For roughly half the women sharing a household meant discontinuing a

pattern of living alone, after several decades. For another large portion, 44 percent, a shared residence in retirement was merely a continuation of habits established in early or mid-adulthood. Living alone, in short, was a choice that few of these never-married women invoked in old age. As long-independent women, they—as a group—wanted to exercise control over the conditions in which they might have to endure physical or financial dependency in their future. Therefore, long ahead of time, they had chosen the people with whom and the place in which they would live out the last third of their lives. (p. 160)

RELATIONSHIPS. Friendship and networking with other single women take up a significant amount of time and provide considerable pleasure and support for many single women, especially those who are voluntarily single. Historical accounts of the roles and work of American women are replete with references to female support networks. A striking example is the Jane Addams–Ellen Starr (founders of Hull House) friendship, which expanded to a large network system over the years (Woloch, 1984). The days of settlement houses and group living of single women are far in the past. However, even though most single women of financial means live alone, strong networks with other women are established from associations in the workplace, church, and other organizations. Writing about single black women, Staples (1981) notes that their friendships with other women serve as both a support and a barrier to successful relationships with black men. Mary Jo, a 35-year-old teacher, differed strongly with Staples's reference to friendships with women thwarting relationships with men. "With the shortage of eligible black men, I would have become a hermit if I didn't have friendships with women, who have interests similar to mine, and with whom I have a good time when we vacation together, and/or have an evening out for dinner or the theater," she exclaimed. She went on to say that her women friends aid and abet each other in their efforts in developing and maintaining a relationship with a man. However, each of them resents being "used as a means to an end if a sister isn't up front with us."

Some reported long-standing platonic relationships with men, who provide emotional support and companionship (especially at those times when a social activity calls for a male escort). These platonic associations may or may not continue after the male friend's marriage or romantic involvement with another woman. However, in most instances known to the writer, such relationships sharply dilute platonic ties.

The relaxation of the code of the double standard of sexual behavior (which dates back to the 1920s, but became more pronounced in the decade of the 1960s) and the easy availability of contraceptive measures allowed single women the freedom to be sexual persons without guilt. Sexual liaisons may involve relatively long-term commitments or may be more numerous and over shorter time frames. However, as in the past, married men are available as sexual partners if single women (or married) should so choose such a relationship. Some who have done so report that such a relationship is preferred because of their preference to be free of a total commitment. In the current era of nationwide concern about sexually transmitted diseases, most single women (who took part in the survey) volunteered that their choices are sharply curtailed. However, even some of the most mature and responsible women admit that they are not consistent in the practice of "safe sex."

Some single women come to settle for the kind of intimate relationships that Lurie, in the novel *Foreign Affairs* (1984), describes as the lot for "plain women": "far more often, she must relax her requirements for commitment, constancy and romantic passion; she must cease to hope for declaration of love, admiring stares. . . . They often have a sex life. What they lack, rather, is a love life" (p. 14).

Some single women are very much a part of their families of origin or a family developed by "adoption." A close relationship with the wife or husband of a nonrelative family may have been established years before the marriage, and both partners and children are comfortable in viewing the nonrelative single woman as an integral member of the family. She knows that she can be included in family gatherings and celebrations, but the need for privacy (the single women's and the family's) and involvement in other activities is respected. Expectations from one's family and segments of the broader society vary. If the single woman has achieved a higher socioeconomic status than that of other members of her family of origin, she may be expected to be able to "help out" when relatives are in financial or emotional straits. No matter that a married sibling or a single brother may be in a similar or even better position to be of assistance, it is not unusual for the first "cry for help" to be directed to the single woman. Should she feel guilty about her success, and a sizable number do, the single woman may be driven to volunteer to "help out"; then, she finds herself trying to submerge the resulting feelings of resentment.

Relationships established with peers and business/professional colleagues can produce both positive and negative sequelae. The friendships that Laura had established with classmates during their years in undergraduate school continued through graduate and law school. Later, some of the group became more involved with various professional organizations and the university alumni association, and relationships became more work-oriented. Laura's unmarried status was viewed as giving her more free time than her married friends, and she was often volunteered by others to take on a specific task or asked to follow up on a matter because a friend, who had assumed a certain responsibility, had to redefine her priorities because of family responsibilities. It was as if it were assumed that Laura had no social life or responsibilities to her family. Susan, a 39-year-old accountant, has become resentful in response to similar experiences. Unlike Laura, Susan covets marriage and adapts to singleness less well each year. Bouts of depression about her state prompted her to seek professional help.

Is LONELINESS A PROBLEM? Adams (1976) noted that single persons must come to terms with the possibility of recurrent periods of loneliness in the course of achieving psychological autonomy, a strong factor influencing singleness. However, many single people are apparently immune to loneliness or are very successful in warding it off. They may live alone, but they are not isolated. They are often alone, but they do not experience loneliness. Usually, these women have a number of meaningful attachments, including family, friends, lovers, and/or business/professional associates. Some work hard at developing and maintaining these relationships; for others, the contacts just seem to happen.

Loneliness was indeed a problem for Susan, the accountant previously mentioned. Not so for a 30-year-old attorney, who hopes to make a career in international law. She expressed an opinion that everyone has moments of loneliness, but she has never viewed it to be a problem. Her social life paralleled that of many others in the survey; that is, she's on good terms with family members, with whom she has ongoing contacts, and can "count on" a number of close friends. Most of the professional women in the survey were involved with a specific activity of their respective professional organizations, an activity which they enjoyed and which took up a significant period of time at frequent intervals. However, some of the women in the sample experienced oppressive loneliness when they arrived at a couple-oriented social gathering without an escort. A 45-year-old pediatrician recounted such experiences during a 3-year stint in her first full-time faculty position. As a newcomer to the university and to the city, she looked forward to the first faculty social, but she was not prepared for the "cold shoulders" shown by a sizable number of the wives of her colleagues. Later, she learned that she had been identified as a *femme fatale*. Janet was chagrined to learn that she had been so identified, especially since she had always been highly competitive with her peers—male and female—and was totally career-oriented. Janet's experiences are not unusual among young and middle-aged single women. Unlike single men, unmarried women are not as sought after to attend a gathering of couples; "the extra man" is welcomed, but not so the "extra woman."

Loneliness was identified as a significant problem for several of the interviewees who immigrated to the United States in their early adult years. Culture shock appears to have been a factor in promoting isolation and ensuing loneliness. So it was for a 33-year-old Filipino, who has earned a degree in journalism but has been unable to find a job in her field. The loneliness seeded in homesickness was probably compounded for this young woman, and other of her Filipino women friends, by the fact that they had not found positions in the fields for which they were trained.

Dunn and Dunn (1980) have written of the loneliness rooted in racial discrimination. They note that "many Black workers hired to work in the virgin territory of white corporations and institutions have gained [only] marginal positions in the social networks of the dominant group" (p. 295). Feelings of alienation and loneliness are strong ripple effects. For a number of black women in the sample populations, the position of marginality and feelings of loneliness were rooted in the workplace. Evelyn, an associate dean at a prestigious university, was the only black female educator appointed to a national committee that was developed to discuss and plan for substantive changes in secondary education curricula. During the course of the deliberations, her comments were ignored for the most part. However, there were a number of instances wherein another member offered a suggestion that paralleled the one she had put forth previously. It was obvious that she had been heard but was to receive no credit for her contributions, an experience cited by many women, regardless of their marital status, race, or ethnicity. For Evelyn the exclusionary process extended to the social scene. Invitations to join the group for dinner and/or a "nightcap" were ambiguous, or she was not asked to participate. It should be noted that singleness, as related to marital status, was not the issue, but the fact that she was the single person that was different from the group because of her racial identity. However, there were other occasions when Evelyn felt that she was in a position of triple jeopardy (as related to her gender, racial identity, and unmarried status), and this compounded the feelings of loneliness in the couple-oriented social gatherings of members of her department. Not infrequently, the bottled-up anger and depression impedes her functioning. Evelyn's experiences are known to be commonplace among achieving, single black women.

A sizable number of women reported considerable success in their efforts to combat loneliness. For years, 50-year-old Karen, a physician, and a single woman colleague planned a yearly vacation around the Christmas holidays. Of course, it was their good fortune to be financially secure and to engage in work that allowed them this kind of time off. Another single woman, less well off financially, and several close women friends (all single) planned a pot-luck dinner for family-oriented holidays and some activity (a concert, theater) for Saturday nights. The size of the group varied from time to time. Several of the women were involuntarily single, and it was understood that their acceptance of a date with a prospective mate would not meet with the group's disfavor. Concert series, church or synagogue, and professional organizational activities also provided opportunities that served to guard against loneliness. Family activities were listed as significant factors for many women. For the past 30 years, 60-year-old Beth has been included in the family activities of a sister and brother-in-law; she continues to be considered an integral member of this family unit, which has expanded with the marriages of the now-adult children and their offspring. Sarah, an executive secretary in a prestigious law firm, has had similar experiences with an "adopting" family (the husband and children of a good friend of long standing).

MOTHERHOOD. A growing number of single women in their 30s are choosing to become mothers. The lessening of the stigma of having children out of wedlock and the advent of the new reproductive methods, as well as the changes in adoption policies, widen the opportunities for parenting by single persons. Some women are impregnated by partners they choose to be a willing father; others decide to carry an unplanned pregnancy to term. Marriage is not considered; in fact, the function of motherhood is viewed as distinctly separate from the function of wife (Hunter College Women's Studies Collective, 1983).

Respondents to an inquiry directed to 4,900 career women included 20% who answered that they conceived and delivered their babies out of wedlock (McKaughan & Kagan, 1986). A 30-year-old single social worker stated her desire and commitment to have a baby. She saw her biological clock as a time bomb. A 37-year-old single school counselor wrote of her struggle to achieve motherhood (Walker, 1985). Her initial efforts focused on adoption, but she was turned down by a private agency on the basis that she did not have enough money. Yet a public agency offered her the possibility of adopting a handicapped child or a teenager. After being turned down when she sought to adopt a child from another country, she followed the advice of a physician who suggested artificial insemination. This single mother was not blinded to possible difficulties that might develop (e.g. the child's questions about his father's identity) but was prepared to deal with them. Time will tell. The passage of time will also provide opportunities for researchers to identify and evaluate the consequences of the new reproductive technologies.

Elsie was in her 32nd year when she became pregnant. Although the pregnancy was unplanned, she never considered abortion or adoption; in fact, she severed the relationship with the man she was dating when he urged her to have an abortion. Elsie has always seen herself as an independent person and had no qualms about supporting herself and her child. In fact, she plans to expand her family by adopting a child. In looking back, she recalls that she always wanted to have children but had focused on foster parenting or adoption. She remains "lukewarm about marriage; would consider it if the right man came along, although I'm not looking."

SUMMARY STATEMENT

The heterogeneity of several groups of never-married women has been discussed in terms of classification, living styles, and problems said to be of particular concern to this varied population. The women described were fortunate to have been well educated and middle class, whether by birth or by acquisition. Unlike their less well-educated and economically secure sisters, they have many choices that lead to their well-being.

A cursory review of the images of singleness, as depicted by the broader society, revealed the continuation of negativity about single women in many circles—this in spite of the fact that the numbers of unmarried women are increasing and they are finding greater acceptance. As illustrated by a number of women surveyed, singleness does not serve as a barrier in obtaining benefits that once were available through marriage: financial security, satisfying relationships, children. Another story is told by single women who long to be married.

Regardless of their classification, many single women are subjected to discrimination—economic and social. The development of and involvement in networking have been instrumental in warding off and combating any untoward effects related to being single.

REFERENCES

Adams, M. (1976). *Single blessedness: Observations on the single status in married society.* New York: Basic Books.

Dunn, E. F., & Dunn, P. C. (1980). Loneliness and the black experience. In J. Hartog, J. R. Audy, and Y. A. Cohen (Eds.), *The anatomy of loneliness* (pp. 284–302). New York: International Universities Press.

Hunter College Women's Studies Collective. (1983). *Women's realities, women's choices.* New York: Oxford University Press.

Lurie, A. (1984). *Foreign affairs.* New York: Avon Books.

McKaughan, M., & Kagan, J. (1986). The mother plunge: The real truth about having—or not having—a baby from 4,900 career women who know. *Working Woman, 1,* 69.

Simon, B. L. (1987). *Never married women.* Philadelphia: Temple University Press.

Staples, R. (1979). The myth of black macho: A response to angry feminists. *Black Scholar,* March–April.

Staples, R. (1981). *The world of black singles.* Westport, CT: Greenwood Press.

Stein, P. J. (1976). *Single.* Englewood Cliffs, NJ: Prentice-Hall.

Walker, S. (1985). Why I became a single mother. *Ladies Home Journal, 1,* 22.

Woloch, N. (1984). Women and the American experience. New York: Knopf.

Chapter 3

Foster Families: The Demands and Rewards of Being a Foster Mother

PAUL M. FINE AND MARY PAPE

Love is the voice under all silences,
the hope which has no opposite in fear

CUMMINGS, 1965, p. 158

Willingness to parent other people's children is one of our better human qualities. During 1982, in the United States, at least 425,000 children and adolescents lived in foster homes under public supervision (Edna McConnell Clark Foundation, 1985). Providing foster parenting to young people whose family relationships have been disrupted is a demanding task that will not appeal to every family. Nevertheless, for certain individuals, being a foster parent is uniquely rewarding.

The authors of this chapter, a special educator and a child psychiatrist, have collaborated with hundreds of foster homes, many continuously over the course of 15 years and most from the same relatively stable midwestern community. Foster parents usually bring children to us with physical-medical, educational, and mental health problems. Typical cases also involve family stress, placement complications, and traumatic development. It is from clinical experience with foster children treated comprehensively that we offer a perspective on foster parenting.

The foster care system is complex and heterogeneous. Legally, foster parents are less protected than adoptive parents. Emotionally, foster homes are more engrossing than group homes or institutions. In view of pressures inherent to foster care, potential foster mothers are well advised to become informed before accepting children. Important considerations include characteristics of children and adolescents who are available for placement, characteristics of families whose children are

PAUL M. FINE • Creighton-Nebraska Universities Department of Psychiatry, Omaha, Nebraska 68108.   MARY PAPE • Iowa Western Community College, Council Bluffs, Iowa 51502.

placed, foster home licensing, agency procedures, the effects of foster parenting on foster families, and qualities that appear to insulate foster families from stress. Some of the realities of foster parenting are presented in this chapter. Case descriptions are used throughout the chapter to convey actual situations, but details have been changed to ensure confidentiality.

FOSTER CHILDREN

Children and adolescents usually enter foster care by court orders, the vast majority of which are made for three reasons: mental incapacity of a parent or guardian, unmanageable behavior by a child or adolescent, and protection from abuse or neglect. Other reasons for placement relate to infants and children whose physical-medical or developmental problems require skilled family care. Two or more reasons generally coexist in any particular case (Fanshel, 1982; Kliman, Schaeffer, & Friedman, 1982).

Overriding goals of the court for children in placement center around legal, physical, and emotional protection, and permanency. Social services are assigned to state, county, and private agencies as necessary to achieve the court's goals. The preferred outcome of foster placement in our society is a quick return of the child to an improved birth family. Failing a return home, legal termination of parental rights may be sought to free the child for adoption. Failing adoption, stable, ongoing care in a specialized foster home, group home, or institution usually is a last resort (Maluccio & Fein, 1983).

In theory, foster placements are benign, time-limited, once-in-a-lifetime events during which the foster home is well supported, the child's developmental needs met, progress carefully monitored, siblings kept together, birth parents offered appropriate services, and court decisions toward permanency efficiently accomplished.

Yet serious defects in all aspects of the foster care system have been identified by several large-scale studies (Children's Defense Fund, 1978; Gruber, 1978; National Commission on Children in Need of Parents, 1979; Shyne & Schroeder, 1978; Vinokur-Kaplan & Hartman, 1986). The disparity between the ideal and the reality of our system is demonstrated by the typical child in foster care. Statistically, he or she is 11 years old, has been in the system about 5 years, has lived in two or more foster homes, has little contact with birth parents or caseworkers, and is not free for adoption (Fanshel, 1982; Shyne & Schroeder, 1978). Crucial decisions concerning child care thus may occur randomly or fall to foster parents by default, without the security of legal custody.

Fostering Abused Children

Abused children in emergency and other temporary placements create a distinct set of pressures for foster mothers. Benny's story is a case in point. At age 8, Benny was picked up by the Child Protective Services. A teacher reported facial bruises, which Benny said had been inflicted by his father. Further investigation found the boy living with his father, age 38, a 22-year-old stepmother, an 11-year-old birth sister, and 8-year-old twin stepbrothers. Benny's birth mother had disappeared from his life when he was 2. Her whereabouts were unknown. His father, who worked part time repairing trucks, had a history of arrests for burglary. Conditions in the home were described as marginal. Benny was placed in an emergency foster home.

Psychiatric evaluation was sought by the caseworker at the foster mother's request. The foster mother had noted that Benny cried for no apparent reason, ate compulsively, followed her around incessantly, and aggressively bothered female foster siblings. Once, he said in frustration, "Nobody loves me but God." The foster mother described Benny as preoccupied with nudity and eager to start conversations about adult sexual activities. She and the caseworker were concerned that Benny might be sent back to an abusive situation. They hoped the psychiatrist could document reasons for continued protection.

During a psychiatric interview Benny was shy and guarded. He had an oppressed, "hang-dog," slouched posture. Although Benny spoke and acted immaturely, he was well oriented, only mildly depressed, and able to respond thoughtfully to questions. Anxiety and insecurity during the interview appeared to stem from dysfunctional attachments and abuse. For example, Benny identified his foster mother as "my real mother," yet he had known her for only 10 days. In contrast, he referred to his stepmother as "my fake mother," asserting that she was inconsequential in his life. Benny's most consistent relationship appeared to be with his father, toward whom he expressed ambivalent fear and hatred. At one point in the interview, Benny lifted his shirt, revealing several well-defined scars, which he said were the result of whippings, beatings, and burnings by his father. Asked to draw a picture of his father, Benny produced "my father" as "Dracula," replete with black eyes, sharp teeth, "angry mouth," beard, mustache, and pointed "Dracula hands" (see Figure 1). While drawing, he detailed physical abuse but denied sexual abuse. Rather, there was evidence of indirect overstimulation. For example, when asked to describe his parent's relationship, he matter-of-factly responded, "They f—k." Benny clearly said he feared to return home and felt safe at the foster home.

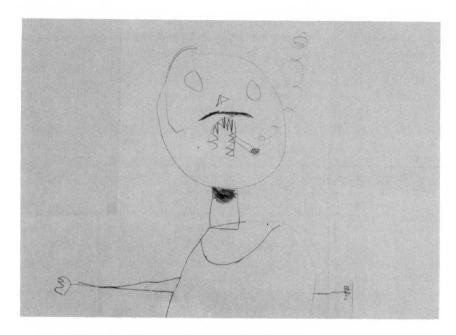

Figure 1. Eight-year-old Benny's drawing of his father as "Dracula."

In light of Benny's evaluation, we recommended ongoing protection in a foster home and continued investigation of the birth family. The evaluation also indicated a need for help with individual problems, including immaturity, hyperalertness, cognitive and social delays, anxiety, rage, and misery.

In this particular case, Benny was spared an immediate return to his abusive father. Yet he was to experience other frustrations within the foster care system. Despite the fact that Benny felt secure at the emergency foster home, they had no room, and he was moved to another family. According to the caseworker, the second set of foster parents reacted punitively, "verging on abuse," when they discovered Benny dressed as a girl playing with their preschool son. Benny then pleaded with the caseworker to take him to her home. She could not, but she was able to find another home for him, this time with a special education teacher who knew Benny and was licensed for foster care.

Thus far, Benny's last placement has been relatively satisfactory for him and his foster mother, but problems persist. Benny's new foster mother is required by court order to drop him off each week at the Welfare Department. There, Benny has brief supervised visits with his father. The visits are awkward and provoke anxiety for all concerned. Litigation is in process. The future is uncertain.

Benny's placements illustrate a frequent emotional dilemma for foster mothers. Courts of law are required to protect children from abuse while at the same time respecting the rights of birth and adoptive families. In cases where the child's rights and the parent's rights are difficult to reconcile, foster parents can find themselves raising children from week to week, for months or years, while the court attempts to reach a decision about the child's future. Naturally, loving foster mothers become attached to children even in the most ambiguous situations. Unfortunately, court decisions affirming legal rights for foster parents have been few and far between (Ordway, 1985). Thus, because their foster children are liable to be sent back to a birth family or a preadoptive home with little or no preparation, the foster family is continually vulnerable to hurt. Nowhere is the dilemma more poignant than for foster parents of toddlers placed as infants and whose primary attachments are to the foster family. However, returning a child or adolescent to birth parents who are inadequate, abusive, or dangerous can be equally difficult.

FOSTERING DISABLED CHILDREN

Physical-medical, psychiatric, and educational problems are more frequent among children and adolescents in the foster care system than in the general population (Swire & Kavaler, 1977). Foster children who are placed specifically for help with disabilities typify the challenge their situation presents. The story of one child, Melissa, exemplifies exceptional parenting for extraordinary problems.

Diane Baumgartner, Melissa's foster and, later, adoptive mother, wrote a book about her experiences with the child. In the book, Baumgartner describes stressful mixed emotions on first encounter with her 7-month-old foster daughter. At the time, Melissa's problems included hydrocephalus, cerebral atrophy, and profound retardation. The infant was blind, functionally deaf, physically weak, and prone to develop infections. She could not turn, kick, or swallow food. Baumgartner (1980) writes: "The lifelessness of her body stunned me. She felt different from any baby I had ever held. Her head was heavier than anticipated, and her arms and legs dangled like a rag doll . . . but looking at the helpless infant in my son's arms caused every mothering instinct I had ever felt to rumble inside me. . . . Maybe I was afraid of becoming more attached than I wanted to be . . . of caring more than I wanted to care" (p. 40).

The book goes on to describe how life with Melissa was built around a routine of special feeding, exercise, sensory stimulation, and training for communication. Surgery for glaucoma became necessary, pneumonia developed, and the Baumgartners nursed the child at home. Gradually, with care, Melissa learned to take pleasure from personal contact with family members, smile with joy, recognize simple signs and signals, and accept comfort. With time, Diane Baumgartner resolved her feelings about Melissa. In conversation, she recalls with wry humor an incident that illustrated Melissa's progress: "Once, in a restaurant, Melissa was with the family, mute, immobile, well-dressed, and happy in a specially molded infant seat. A lady at the next table leaned over to compliment us, saying, 'That's the most well-behaved child I ever saw' " (personal communication, 1980).

Toward the end of Melissa's first year, she was adopted by the Baumgartners. Diane Baumgartner explains: "I wanted Melissa's mother to love her the way we did, but I knew this was unrealistic. She held the baby away from her, down in her lap. She looked at us in astonishment when we took joy in Melissa's appearance. After adoption by us, Melissa's mother was more at ease with her daughter."

Melissa lived for 2 years and 9 months. The Baumgartners comforted her as she died. Then, they comforted members of her family at the funeral. In retrospect, Tony, Diane, and their four sons value the time Melissa spent in the family. Diane says: "Melissa's life was an encouragement to seek worth and value in all people. . . . I learned that you don't have to be afraid to love someone you can't be with forever. . . . We were able to help Melissa's mother feel like a worthwhile parent. . . . As the boys developed pride in our foster children, they lost all concept of the word retarded. To them everyone was smart in his own way."

Over the years, we have encountered other foster mothers who successfully helped children cope with a variety of equally discouraging physical conditions, including juvenile diabetes, epilepsy, cystic fibrosis, terminal leukemia, and Prader-Willi syndrome. In each case, the foster mother had to overcome mixed feelings to care for the child.

BIRTH FAMILIES

Additional pressures for foster mothers arise from the fact that children and adolescents usually come to foster care from homes with severe family problems. Statistically, the average foster child's birth family is headed by a single mother with two or three children. The father is neither available nor supportive. The family is likely to suffer from limited economic resources, undereducation, and higher than average rates for drug and alcohol abuse, mental illness, imprisonment, and transgenerational family violence (Fanshel, 1982; Kliman et al., 1982; Shyne & Schroeder, 1978).

Foster parents tell us that children and adolescents bring family problems to their homes along with the luggage. It is for this reason that many foster parents find it necessary to work with the families of their foster children. Under optimal circumstances, work between birth parents and foster families grows into constructive, extended familylike relationships. When direct contact is limited or absent, information from social services is a useful substitute. Then, relevant information about the birth family enables foster parents to help children cope with reasons for placement, family visits, returning home, and, when necessary, preadoptive replacement.

FOSTERING WITH THE HELP OF A BIRTH MOTHER

Danny's story illustrates how a skillful foster mother helped a displaced adolescent and his mother to find inner strength to reconcile. The story, one of several successful efforts by this particular mother, is presented in detail to illustrate how serious problems were overcome through her work with the family. Danny was born a healthy, well-endowed infant, but he was removed from his mother's home as ungovernable by the time he was 5. Problems at the time included defiance toward adults; competitiveness with peers; fondling female playmates; a need to control, aggravate, and agitate others; poor frustration tolerance; and destructiveness with toys. He also exhibited frantic nervous overactivity that alternated with compliance, charm, and creative expressions of inborn talent. A psychologist who tested him noted evidence of overstimulation, which was thought related to having observed adult sexual activity. The psychologist reported:

> This examiner has never obtained a drawing of a man from a five-year-old like this one. The head is extremely small, which is not what one expects from the drawing of a younger child, and the body was over-emphasized, being probably a third of the paper. The drawing was nude with the bellybutton and penis drawn. When Danny drew the penis, he glanced up at the examiner to see what reaction he might observe. This is not the type of drawing one expects from a five or six year old child. Generally, one expects more emphasis on the head and intellectual functions, rather than the body and physical functions.

In retrospect, Danny's mother, Belle, described her son's first 5 years in terms of loving care alternating with chaos. Bright and pretty, but immature, she married at 17 to get away from home, gave birth to Danny and a younger brother, and was divorced. Then, in quick succession, her parents divorced, her mother moved to another state, she lost custody of her younger son to his father, and her father married a woman close to Belle's age. Often, in those days, Belle and Danny lived with a variety of relatives and lovers, "from hand to mouth." Just before

Danny's removal, Belle became addicted to hard drugs. Deeply attached to her son, she concealed the addiction and resisted efforts by the state to terminate parental rights.

Danny spent the middle years of his childhood in a variety of foster and group homes. Visits with members of his extended family, while frequent and meaningful, also were unpredictable and painful. Danny's birth father showed little interest. His mother remained disorganized. Generally, the boy performed adequately at school but protested miserably at home in each placement. By the time he was 9, his behavior had become so unmanageable that he was psychiatrically hospitalized, then placed long term in a semiinstitutional children's home. When Danny was 12, a caseworker helped his mother find services to get her addiction under control. Belle, then 30, experienced success and said she wanted Danny back. The caseworker moved Danny to a transitional foster home and arranged for psychiatric and family services.

Despite everyone's efforts, progress toward reunification was minimal that year. Belle seemed overwhelmed by the intricacies of setting up family housekeeping. In desperation she moved in with her father but soon rediscovered how bad she felt when he became domineering, drunk, and verbally abusive. Now, Belle also found it difficult to cope with a young stepmother, a 9-year-old half brother, and the boarder. In an attempt to bolster finances toward independence, she accepted night work as a bar waitress. The job required absence from home in the evenings and sleeping days. Belle knew she would be under additional stress. She asked Danny for understanding and patience, explaining that her schedule would be more manageable once they got established. Regrettably, Danny could not respond positively to his mother's plea to help. He was pubescent, preoccupied, and could muster little understanding or patience. Rather, he expressed overt contempt, anger, and disillusionment over what he felt was Belle's "failures and excuses."

Inevitably Danny's negative attitude became directed toward the foster family in the foster home. Unfortunately, these particular foster parents had little patience, with either Danny or his mother. The situation deteriorated, and it was only a matter of time before they asked Danny to leave. The "last straw" was to find Danny training a neighbor's German shepherd dog to attack their children. Now Danny and Belle both experienced despair. Desperately, he demanded that his mother relinquish parental rights, explaining that he wanted to be adopted by someone else in order to "live a normal life." Reluctantly, Belle agreed. Once again the caseworker overcame numerous practical obstacles, located a preadoptive home, and arranged for Danny's placement.

The preadoptive mother was single, 39, successful, career-oriented, and secretly gay. Her home was well organized. She and Danny traveled. She taught him to drive, fish, and hunt, and he liked life with her. However, to the surprise and chagrin of his mother-to-be, as Danny became more attached, he also became more possessive, controlling, restrictive, hostile and easily frustrated. "Perhaps," she thought, "he is not the son of my dreams," and she began to regret the decision to adopt him. Then, following an incident during which Danny physically intruded on her love life, she abandoned him.

At the age of 13, Danny once again found himself in foster placement, but this time at the home of Margaret and Al Martinez, a long-married couple in their late 40s. Biologically childless, the Martinezes enjoyed raising other people's teenage boys in their large, rambling frame house. Margaret and Al were respected in the neighborhood. They maintained good working relationships with schools, agencies, psychotherapists, and other professionals in the community. Their home was well established and smoothly organized. Most important for Danny's future, they lived near his original home. Margaret knew Danny's family, had watched Belle grow up, and understood their family's limitations. Danny fit in with the other four Martinez foster sons, and they determined to stand behind him.

Margaret defined Danny's problems as follows: "Nature dealt Danny adequate cards [with which to play the game of life], but he insists on gambling recklessly [with fate]." In fact, Danny was developing into a handsome, bright, athletic, adolescent. He was in many ways a natural leader but was frequently depressed or self-centered and lacked judgment. For example, that year he organized his foster brothers to play Frisbee with shingles pried from the Martinez roof, threw rocks at cars from the highway overpass, helped start a fire at the local ice cream shop, got suspended from school, and became involved in neighborhood brawls. Margaret helped Danny work his way out of each difficulty. Stubbornly, he refused to acknowledge her help. Then, as if to create more distance, he pressured the caseworker for another chance at adoption. Doggedly, the caseworker prevailed upon Belle's older sister to give Danny a try on their family farm.

Margaret Martinez was hurt and disappointed but not deterred by Danny's defection. She wished Danny success in his new home yet assured him he could return if necessary. Again, perhaps predictably, Danny's self-defeating pattern prevailed. The adoption fell through and with it the farm placement. However, now Danny requested a return to the Martinez family. He agreed to cooperate with the rules of their home and to respect Belle, his birth mother. Belle, in turn, made herself available to help. At last, the cycle of failure and rootlessness was interrupted.

Supportive psychotherapy resumed while Danny was at the Martinez home. One day, during a session, he presented the therapist with a mask he had constructed at school. The mask had small, pinched features, which the boy appeared to view with a mixture of anxiety and disgust. Danny explained that the mask represented his old, constricted self, then asked to have it stored at the therapist's office. A photograph of Danny's mask is shown in Figure 2.

About a month later, Danny presented the therapist with another construction, a life-size, two-dimensional representation of what he said was his ideal self. The portrait boasted clean-cut and open features, sporty clothes, and a rebel flag above the heart. A head-and-shoulders photograph of Danny's self-portrait is shown in Figure 3. The disparity between Danny's inner feelings and his ideal self-image is apparent from his art work. The challenge for adequate care by Margaret is implicit.

During the next 3 years, with Margaret's help, Danny experienced a variety of successes at the Martinez home. He learned family skills and

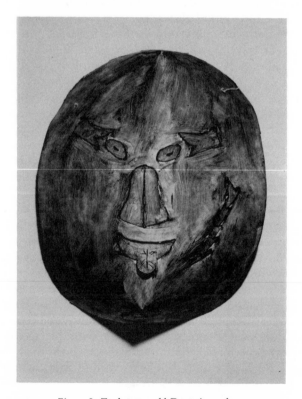

Figure 2. Twelve-year-old Danny's mask.

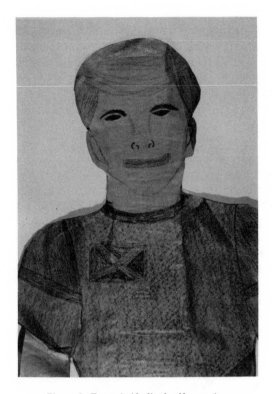

Figure 3. Danny's idealized self-portrait.

developed respect, loyalty, and affection for Margaret, then for Al, and, finally, for his foster siblings. School attendance improved, and Danny channeled excess energy into Tai-Kwan-Do lessons. Also, he behaved more benignly toward Belle, his birth mother.

Belle, as well as Danny, came to rely on Margaret for advice. Among the issues that Belle discussed with Margaret were how to parent effectively, limit setting, finding and keeping a job, balancing a checkbook, organizing a home, and maintaining discretion in intimate affairs. Gradually, Belle achieved a better relationship with her extended family. She found regular work, established a residence, renewed contact with her younger son, and became seriously involved with a dependable, divorced man. Danny saw his mother progress, and he was able to view her in a more positive, new light. Their relationship improved, as did his self-respect. Toward the end of his 16th year, Danny returned to live with Belle.

Now 17, Danny has grown to resemble the exaggerated, idealized self-portrait he produced 4 years earlier. Problems continue. At times, they are severe but no longer seem insurmountable. Danny is hopeful about the future. He takes pride in athletic trophies, spends time with friends, dates occasionally, and is unwavering in his conviction that his mother should buy him a car. Danny and Belle both maintain a relationship with Margaret and Al Martinez, upon whom they call for help when under stress. At Margaret's insistence, Danny and Belle also have continued sessions with the psychiatrist.

Stories similar to those of Danny, Belle, and the Martinez family are frequent among experienced foster parents. They reflect a trend in the social welfare literature to facilitate the integration of birth parents into the helping process (Bryce & Lloyd, 1981; Horejsi, Bertsche, & Clark, 1981; Sinanoglu & Maluccio, 1981). Of course, not all foster children desire reunification or even contact with birth parents, and not all birth parents are receptive to help. We have known terrible situations when babies were kidnapped, death threats were made, and children described orgies of ritual abuse involving birth parents. Under such destructive circumstances, sensible foster parents justifiably demand anonymity or protection. Then, common sense dictates that attempts to help or control the birth family are best conducted away from the foster home.

THERAPEUTIC FOSTER PARENTING

Lynette's story illustrates therapeutic aspects of foster care for a severely traumatized child who was obsessed by memories of her birth mother but unable to return to the biological home. In this instance, the foster mother found it necessary to work closely with a variety of professional and other supportive resources.

Lynette was removed from her mother's custody at the age of 8. Reasons for removal included severe neglect and incestuous abuse. At the time, Lynette was living with her mother, a maternal grandmother, and a 12-year-old sister. The girls' fathers were unknown. Their mother was a marginal individual who suffered episodes of emotional decompensation, engaged in binges of substance abuse, and was herself the victim of childhood sexual abuse. Because Lynette's background and problems were severe, the caseworker placed her with experienced foster parents, Phil and Marie Holland.

As expected, in common with other severely abused, neglected, and sexually misused children, Lynette presented Marie Holland with an array of difficult emotions and behaviors. Predominantly, Lynette's mental state was untrusting, restless, and fearful. She lied and stole from other children in the home and at school. Her sleep was disturbed. She reported frightening nightmares, wet the bed, masturbated compulsively, and often was provocative, aggressive, and agitated. Occasionally, she reached a point of uncontrolled panic or physical assault, "biting and scratching like a cornered little animal." Unpredictably, at other times, Lynette was shy and miserably unhappy, clinging to her foster mother, or withdrawing from all contact. Fortunately, Lynette also had distinct personal assets. She could be affectionate, was eager to please, possessed good native intelligence, and learned quickly with help. However, because Lynette required almost constant attention, she had few friends and often was in trouble at school or on the school bus. Moreover, even when she was happy, Lynette could not acknowledge or integrate previous episodes of troublesome behavior.

Figure 4 is one of several sketches Lynette frantically produced later, during a psychotherapy session. During that particular session, Lynette exhibited overt sexual posturing, whispered memories of painful assault by adult men, and huddled for comfort in Marie Holland's lap. Taken in context, Lynette's sketch is presented to illustrate her pathetically immature, eroticized, distorted self-image, and the challenge it presented to her foster mother.

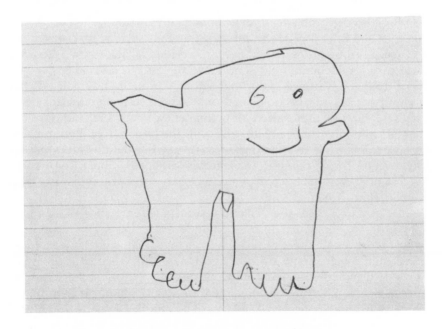

Figure 4. Nine-year-old Lynette's pathetic sketch.

Lynette's disability and Marie Holland's approach to habilitation can be understood in terms of posttraumatic stress disorders. The literature indicates that certain individuals are profoundly influenced by overwhelming social/environmental experiences. Chronically traumatic conditions have been demonstrated to have adverse effects on neurobiological, neurotransmitter, emotional, cognitive, and family development. Behavioral and psychiatric phenomena related to traumatic development include clumsiness, hypervigilance, subtle neurologic dysfunction, biphasic panic-depression responses to stress, intrusive traumatic mental imagery, affect flooding, cognitive inflexibility, conscienceless behaviors, multiple personality phenomena, and borderline personality disorders.

The same literature suggests that corrective primary social experiences can modify the disabling symptoms of overwhelming abuse. Techniques that have been applied directly to the problem include reparenting; unlearning learned helplessness; achieving social, cognitive, and emotional competence; and developing abilities for relaxation and self-expression. Techniques that have been used to facilitate corrective experiences include family therapy, supportive psychotherapy, and certain specific pharmacotherapies (Bretherton & Waters, 1985; Eth & Pynoos, 1985; Goldfarb, 1945; Grabe & Reitnauer, 1985; Kluft, 1986; Rutter, 1971; Triseliotis, 1980; Van Der Kolk, 1987).

Because the problems of developmentally traumatized children are complex and interdependent, intensive settings such as specialized foster homes, group homes, and long-term residential institutions often are necessary for adequate treatment. Nevertheless, specialized foster care has a unique advantage over other settings for many traumatized children. Specifically, foster homes are able to offer corrective social experiences in a natural atmosphere of permanency, family life, and developmental continuity for the child, and with the birth family. Pressures on foster parents while treating these cases are self-evident. For this reason, well-trained foster parents, manageable caseloads, and case-oriented professional backup are considered necessary for success (Bryant, 1980; Kliman et al., 1982).

In Lynette's case, the Hollands participated in a specialized foster care program, in which foster parents are therapists and support is provided by regular peer group meetings that also include a caseworker and a child psychiatrist (Christensen & Fine, 1979). Within this program, Marie Holland constructed a network of services specific for Lynette's special needs. She hired and trained a college student to help in the home, scheduled psychiatric sessions, and enrolled Lynette in a highly structured school program. As experienced foster parents, the Hollands also were able to call upon an ongoing personal network of professional support, which included a pediatrician, a dentist, a lawyer, caseworkers, mental health professionals, special educators, and community self-help agencies for alcoholics, incestuous families, and the mentally ill. In addition, Phil and Marie were members of a regional foster and adoptive parents' club through which they maintained social contacts, compared notes with other parent-therapists, and advocated for better conditions.

Perhaps, the most important network of support for Marie Holland and other foster mothers is family and close friends. In this instance, with the help of her husband, Marie was able to motivate their other children to accept Lynette into the home. Also, with her help, the family tolerated occasional visits by Lynette's mother who, in turn, responded constructively. Then, for the first time, Lynette's mother faced the fact that Lynette was a victim of sexual abuse, resisted family pressures to return her daughter to an abusive situation, and, ultimately, helped with the girl's recovery. To Marie Holland's satisfaction, Lynette now is secure in their family, where she has made slow but steady progress toward increased social skills, fewer symptomatic expressions of post-traumatic stress, and greater inner security.

FOSTER MOTHERS

Who are the women who are most effective at foster parenting? How do they cope with the accumulated pressures of children coming and going from their homes, exposure to the results of childhood illness, abuse, and neglect, and dangerous or incompetent birth families? How do successful foster mothers hold themselves and their families together?

One way to describe effective foster mothers is with statistics. However, remarkably little research has been done to define competent foster parents, and studies to identify factors that correlate with success in placement have not developed enough for direct application (Carbino, 1980; Goldston, 1982). Nevertheless, several statistical studies are available from which a composite description of typical, well-functioning foster families can be drawn. According to these studies, the typical foster family is blue-collar or clerical, with an annual income of about $20,000. In addition to parents, there are four children in the home, including foster children. The family is headed by a married couple, each of whom is between 35 and 50 years old and has a high school education. The parents are family-oriented and provide foster care because they want children in the home. Their home is well organized and developmentally stimulating (Cautley & Aldridge, 1975; Fanshel, 1982; Goldston, 1982; Kraus, 1971).

Other statistical characteristics of functional foster families are less uniform. For example, a large portion of foster families are headed by members of minority groups, a reflection of the fact that minority group children are overrepresented in the foster care system (Shyne & Schroeder, 1978). Also, many foster families are headed by single women, frequently widows. However, minority and single-parent-headed foster families both appear to resemble the functional group as a whole in terms of economic status, age, family size, and motivation (Goldston, 1982).

From clinical experience with foster care, we believe we can add another perspective on successful foster parents. Without doubt, women usually take the lead in good foster parenting, and those who have mastered the art maintain effective working relationships with other adults in the home, including often, but not always, a husband, grandparents, and grown children. Successful foster mothers are notable for strength of character, personal stability, maturity, and effectiveness. As a group, they are sociable, well organized, loving, realistic, and humane. Most say they enjoy the routine work of making a home and parenting a family with all age groups. Generally, they approach their children's physical, emotional, and behavioral problems with tolerance, as a challenge to help. Typically, they are capable of introspection and have a small circle of close personal friends but also maintain an extensive network of extended family and kinlike relationships. Many are personally religious. Frequently, they participate in organized community activities such as parent-teacher associations, church groups, scouting, and Little League. Out of necessity, successful foster mothers also become adept at relating to social service, school, health, and other bureaucratic systems (Fine, 1985).

As with any group in society, outstanding foster parents do not lack emotional problems. However, on occasions when one or another has consulted us for personal help, the presenting problem almost always was "burnout," a transient episode of stress-related anxiety or depression precipitated by overcommitment or overintensity toward family matters, including foster children. In these instances, most of the foster mothers described motivations to provide foster care in terms of an inner need to actualize deeply held family values. One successful foster mother commented that her parents had provided foster care. She felt she was continuing a family tradition. Another foster mother described how, when her parents died, an aunt had given her and three siblings a home. She felt she was paying back a debt of kindness. For yet another mother, serendipity played a role. She explained: "When our daughter became ill and died, we became involved with social services and mental health professionals. The experience got us out of our small world . . . to . . .

become acquainted with children with special problems. . . . We decided to help them."

Of course, not all foster parents are well motivated. Over the years, we have encountered people who accept foster children in order to satisfy pathological motivations, including pedophilia, unresolved bereavement, alcoholism, and simple greed. However, because the work of foster parenting is so demanding and closely controlled, pathological foster parents usually do not remain long at the task.

DEDICATION TO THE FAMILY. Clinically, the overriding impression concerning successful foster parents is their basic dedication to family life. This sense of dedication includes shared family values, strong leadership, effective commitment, and direct communication. Specifics of family organization and ways of insulating foster families from stress vary from situation to situation, but dedication to the family and its values consistently underlie daily life in successful foster homes.

An example of the commitment and stability of one foster family is reflected by a note written by a 13-year-old girl to her foster mother. The note also reflects how matter-of-factly this displaced teenager perceives her foster mother's compassion and good humor in dealing with down-to-earth, here-and-now developmental issues.

> This I guaranty that I positively will promise that I will try to remember to clean up the hair in the sink and try not bite my fingernails and remember to hang up my robe. And I will remember to feed and water Shaderack and try to remember to unload the dishwasher every night and afternoon. This is a promise I will always keep. This guaranty will last the whole year, and through March, April, May and June and the rest of the year I will try and always do the things I'm supposed to do. And if I am away or anywhere else, I will remember to do these things, and be polite and have my very best manners. Because when I eat at the table I am a bit nervous and my hands get a little bit shaky. I really don't know why they shake, but maybe it's because I'm trying not to make my food spill off and make a fool out of myself and make Sherry, Rita, Mary Beth, and Bill and you uncomfortable. And it makes me uncomfortable too when I am eating at the table. But, I didn't tell you this, every night when I pray, I also pray for God to help me so I could be better and do what I am supposed to do. And I also pray for you, and Bill, and Sherry, Rita, Mary Beth and Billie because I love you all so much I really don't want anything to happen to any of you! And also my real family! And if you feel sad, I will try to cheer you up. It doesn't matter if your not my family I still care about you all!
>
> There are some things I don't understand. Like why do girls wear so much make-up. But I think that I won't wear gobs of make-up when I grow up. Because some isn't really good to your skin. I was wondering if you could put a perm in my hair. But I really think I could wait until April. I wish I could tell you straight out. It wouldn't make any sense any way. All that I would say would be like, "Well, I absolutely will promise you I will do my things I'm supposed to do for you! I could tell you better on a piece of white paper with blue skinny lines and a margin. If I had to go anywhere else, I would want to

stay there! Your like a real mom to me, youre nice, you talk like you really
mean it. And you give me the punishment I really need I can't thank you
ever enough to let me come and live with you and your family!

A sense of the skill, vocation, optimism, and patience that goes into
successful foster parenting also is conveyed in an essay by a master
foster mother.

Being a foster parent is: Caring enough to fight the school system to keep a
child back a year in school because you know he can't make the next grade,
and pushing to get another child up a grade because an 11-year-old should
not be in third grade with 8-year-olds, when you know that the child can
make it if given the chance; learning to mother a foster child's mother when
you are not old enough to have a child that age; knowing the frustration of
caring for a child who will drive a nail through the caps on a carton of soft
drinks and then turn the bottles upside down and let the liquid run on the
floor; having your heart turn a flop when you have seen your 8-year-old
return from school wearing your wedding and engagement rings; knowing
the heartache of watching a child's silent tears day after day and being helpless to take the hurt away—maybe in time, but not today.

Being a foster parent is the anxiety of dealing with a seven-year-old who
wants to kill himself because he doesn't want to go live with his mother;
trying to tell a nine-year-old, who has been in foster care since the age of two
and has had little contact with his home, what a real mom is. All of the other
foster kids have a second mom, why doesn't he?

Being a foster parent is rewarding in many ways. It's the job of seeing
tears turn into smiles and laughter, the satisfaction of seeing fits of rage turn
toward a more acceptable form of behavior, the beauty of a withdrawn child
learning to communicate, and helping a child like himself for what he is. It's
hearing the delight of "I did it; I did it" from a child who has just accomplished riding a bike when everyone said it couldn't be done because of
motor problems. It's the privilege of sharing a child's love or earning their
trust, knowing they are returning home better than when they came. It's
helping a child out of a world of fantasy into the world of reality and having a
biological mother say "thank you" for caring for her child when she couldn't.
It's a feeling of being high with no bad effects.

Sure, there is a tug at your heart strings when the three-year-old you got
as a baby goes back to his parents for the last time. You wonder if he'll be
okay, will they take good care of him? Love him as you do? But, you hold
back the tear or let it slide slowly down your cheek and quietly ask God to
watch over the little guy. You tell yourself that there is another child out there
who needs your help for a while, and it helps ease the pain of your present
loss. After all, I have a million dollars worth of memories!

Being a foster parent is the knowledge that, with the help of many
others, you have had a small part in helping a child attain a better, more
normal way of life. At times you wonder if it's worth all the effort, energy,
and sacrifice, and for this foster parent, it is! (Harris, 1980)

Another highly successful foster mother notes that having a large
family helps her cope with the pressures of raising foster children. She
explains, "In a large family all the little things children do can't become

an obsession. The children help each other, and each child has to find a place in everyday living." She goes on to describe how, at first, she experienced worry and guilt toward her birth children because they would have to share the home with a foster child. Then, she recalls with humor, "I realized that I hadn't asked any of my eleven birth children about getting pregnant and thought I also shouldn't have to request their permission to take in foster children. Since the decision by my husband and me to take in the first special needs foster child, we have adopted her and five other hard-to-care-for children. All of our children must accept each other as much as children do in any family."

Most of the birth children from foster families we know complain bitterly about social embarrassment and inconvenience caused by their foster siblings. Nevertheless, almost invariably, the young people also express pride in their parents' altruism, loyalty to the family's values, and protectiveness toward their foster siblings. Most foster mothers believe that the experience with foster siblings has enriched their children's lives.

Essentially, the foster mother's task of personal and family protection is developmental and integrative, often intangible, and sometimes ephemeral. Frequently, the results of her efforts can be seen most clearly in retrospect. Consider, for example, the following tribute, written to her foster mother, after several helpful but troubled years of care, by a 17-year-old girl.

> My mother Frances a sweet, innocent, kind and important woman in my life. She cared for me when nobody else would and until this day she is still caring and loving me which I think about a lot of times. She really wants to get to know my mother and I'm sure my mother would like to be a good friend of hers. She likes to work problems out by talking and understanding which is the best way. Most of the time she is doing something for us or trying to make us happy. I try to be good so she can trust me but sometimes I slip and she seems to always forgive me.
>
> My Mother Frances who laughs and giggles a lot. It makes me happy to see her pretty smile. She tries to keep that pretty smile but sometimes we make her angry. She is not the kind of lady who likes to fuss all the time. She is a lady of LOVE. So all the rest of you should be ladies of love and I'm sure you'll make a beautiful Mother.

PRACTICAL CONSIDERATIONS. Prospective foster mothers usually hear about foster care through advertising or by word of mouth. In many communities, brief presentations of "Wednesday's Child" are made on television to interest the public in specific children in need of placement. People who become interested then are encouraged to obtain a license, contact sponsoring agencies, and consider appropriate foster children for placement.

Licensing to do foster care is arranged on a state-by-state basis.

Typical requirements for licensing include good health, freedom from child abuse or felony convictions, and an inspection of the home to ensure certain standards for cleanliness, space, and fire safety. Many licensing departments conduct training sessions. Typically, they orient new foster parents to state policies concerning foster homes, including basic child care, acceptable methods for discipline, and paperwork preparation. Some licensing departments also conduct or sponsor training sessions about child and family development, problems typical of foster care, therapeutic techniques, and cultural sensitivity (Hampson, 1985). In many states, annual license renewal and continuing education are required. Also, limits may be placed on the number of children in any category of foster home, including family group, emergency respite, and long-term homes.

Licensed foster parents may choose from a variety of sponsoring agencies to locate children for placement. Although agencies vary from state to state, some generalizations concerning the type of children they sponsor are possible. For example, private agencies frequently place infants and young children temporarily until an adoptive home can be arranged. County and court programs usually place children and adolescents from homes where there has been serious abuse or neglect. These cases often are in crisis. In contrast, many state and private agencies, including health-oriented agencies, sponsor special-needs children in long-term placement.

Experienced foster parents usually accept children and adolescents from more than one agency, and many also adopt. Under favorable circumstances, careful stepwise matching between foster child and foster home is arranged before the child enters the foster home, and the foster parents participate in subsequent planning by the agency on behalf of the child.

Most states offer foster parents a basic stipend of between $150 and $250 per month for each child. Supplementary payments can be added to the basic stipend when extraordinary care is necessary. The highest amount we know of was $1,500 to care for a terminally ill child. Additionally, medical, dental, and educational costs usually are covered by state or federal funds. Certainly, however, most foster parents do not take in children for the money. Rather, as a medical student remarked, "Foster care is the prototype for not-for-profit cottage industries."

CONCLUSION

It is a paradox, but good foster mothers are far from universally appreciated. At first glance, most people view foster care as a symptom of family disruption rather than one of its solutions. Important recent federal reforms affecting the foster care system rightly emphasize legally permanent homes, preferably with the family of origin. Unfortunately, when reforms such as the federal Indian Child Welfare Act of 1978 and the federal Adoption Assistance and Child Welfare Act of 1980 were enacted, opportunities to reinforce important work by foster families was virtually ignored. For example, positive familylike relationships between foster families and the less fortunate families of their foster children appear to have been overlooked. Consequently, the new federal attention to foster care has been bittersweet for most foster parents. On the one hand, they welcome reform, yet tighter monitoring and control with less support has made creative foster care more difficult.

Almost all women in modern society balance career needs with parenting needs. To one extent or another, they accept or provide substitute care for children. In this context, good foster parents are a scarce but precious social resource, and certain trends in social welfare indicate that more will be needed. Children are the fastest growing population of poor people in the United States. At a rate of 24%, children under the age of 6 experience a higher proportion of poverty than any other age group. Add to this situation the increased number of young people living with one parent, lower wages for women than for men, higher costs for child care, and unemployment or underemployment in families of the children most at risk, and it becomes apparent that more and better services of all types, including foster care, will be required in the future (Children's Defense Fund, 1987).

In the final analysis, the social significance of effective foster mothers transcends government and job requirements. At best, they represent the portion of society for whom skills at childrearing and family life are most highly developed. It is for this reason that good foster mothers make a significant contribution to society, and the rewards they experience are beyond price, including self-satisfaction, respect, and the affection of those whose lives they have touched.

The 12 successful mothers whose work was described in this chapter represent excellence of care in our particular community. As a group, they have fostered or adopted over 300 children and adolescents, and their work has affected positively the lives of many of the children's relatives. Among this group of foster mothers are single as well as married women, representing a variety of cultures and ethnic minorities. We believe that similarly interested, effective women can be found in any community.

For readers who are interested in learning more about foster parenting, a variety of resources are available. Books, pamphlets, and articles describe basic foster care (Felker, 1974; Littner, 1980; Rutter, 1978), how it feels to be a foster child (Hester & Nygren, 1981), how to organize foster parent associations and support groups (Sprouse, 1984), mental health resources (Grabe & Reitnauer, 1985), and services for sexually abused children (Fine & Carnevale, 1984). In addition, numerous other publications discuss permanency for foster children, including legal issues and work with preadoptive, adoptive, minority, and birth families (Barth, Berry, Carson, Goodfield, & Feinberg, 1986; Edna McConnell Clark Foundation, 1985; Horejsi, 1979; Kessel & Robbins, 1984; Leon, 1979; Maluccio & Sinanoglu, 1981; Metropolitan Court Judges Committee, 1986; Murray, 1983; Pike, Downs, Emlen, Downs, & Case, 1977; Stack, 1985). Resource agencies and self-help groups include American Foster Child Resources, Inc. (P.O. Box 271, King George, VA 22485), the Child Welfare League of America (67 Irving Place, New York, NY 10003), the Family Service Association of America (44 East 23rd Street, New York, NY 10010), and the National Association of Former Foster Children (P.O. Box 169, Bay Ridge Station, Brooklyn, NY 11220).

REFERENCES

Barth, R. P., Berry, M., Carson, M. L., Goodfield, R., & Feinberg, B. (1986). Contributors to dissolution of older-child adoptions. *Child Welfare, 65,* 359–371.

Baumgartner, D. B. (1980). *Melissa: The story of a very special baby.* Elgin, IL: David C. Cook.

Bretherton, I., & Waters, E. (Eds.). (1985). Growing points of attachment theory and research. *Monographs of the Society for Research in Child Development, 50* (1, # 2).

Bryant, B. (1980). *Special foster care: A history and rationale.* Verona, VA: People Places.

Bryce, M., & Lloyd, J. C. (Eds.). (1981). *Treating families in the home: An alternative to placement.* Springfield, IL: Charles C Thomas.

Carbino, R. (1980). *Foster parenting: An updated review of the literature.* New York: Child Welfare League of America.

Cautley, P. O., & Aldridge, M. J. (1975). Predicting success in foster care. *Social Work, 20,* 48–53.

Children's Defense Fund. (1978). *Children without homes: An examination of public responsibility to children in out of home care.* Washington, DC: Author.

Children's Defense Fund. (1987). *A children's defense budget: An analysis of FY 1987 federal budget and children.* Washington, DC: Author.

Christensen, G., & Fine, P. (1979). Corrective socialization in the foster care of children. *Child Psychiatry and Human Development, 10,* 15–34.

Cummings, E. E. (1965). *A selection of poems* (p. 158). New York: Harcourt, Brace & World.

Edna McConnell Clark Foundation. (1985). *Keeping families together: The case for family preservation.* New York: Author.

Eth, S., & Pynoos, R. S. (Eds.). (1985). *Post traumatic stress disorder in children.* Washington, DC: American Psychiatric Press.

Fanshel, D. (1982). *On the road to permanency: An expanded data base for service to children in foster care.* New York: Child Welfare League of America.

Felker, E. H. (1974). *Foster parenting young children: Guidelines from a foster parent.* New York: Child Welfare League of America.

Fine, P. (1985). Clinical aspects of foster care. In J. J. Cox & R. D. Cox (Eds.), *Foster care: Current issues, policies and practices.* Norwood, NJ: Ablex.

Fine, P. & Carnevale, P. (1984). Network aspects of treatment for incestuously abused children. In I. R. Stuart & J. G. Greer (Eds.), *Victims of sexual aggression: Treatment of men, women and children.* New York: Van Nostrand Reinhold.

Goldfarb, W. (1945). Psychological privation in infancy and subsequent adjustment. *American Journal of Orthopsychiatry, 15,* 247–255.

Goldston, J. (1982). The foster parents. In G. W. Kliman, W. K. Gilbert, M. H. Schaeffer, & M. J. Friedman (Eds.), *Preventive mental health services for children entering foster home care.* White Plains, NY: Center for Preventive Psychiatry.

Grabe, P. V., & Reitnauer, P. D. (Eds.). (1985). *Adoption resources for mental health professionals.* Mercer, PA: Childrens Aid Society of Mercer, Pennsylvania.

Gruber, A. R. (1978). *Children in foster care: Destitute, neglected, betrayed.* New York: Human Sciences Press.

Hampson, R. (1985). Foster parent training: Assessing its role in upgrading foster care. In J. J. Cox & R. D. Cox (Eds.), *Foster care: Current issues, policies and practices.* Norwood, NJ: Ablex.

Harris, D. (1980). Thank you for caring. *Proceedings of the tenth annual foster parents training program.* St. Louis: National Foster Parents Resource Center.

Hester, G., & Nygren, B. (1981). *Child of rage.* Nashville: Thomas Nelson.

Horejsi, C. R. (1979). *Foster family care: A handbook for social workers, allied professionals and concerned citizens.* Springfield, IL: Charles C Thomas.

Horejsi, C. R., Bertsche, V. A., & Clark, F. W. (1981). *Social work practice with parents of children in foster care: A handbook.* Springfield, IL: Charles C Thomas.

Kessel, J. A., & Robbins, S. P. (1984). The Indian child welfare act: Dilemmas and needs. *Child Welfare, 63,* 225–232.

Kliman, G. W., Schaeffer, M. H., & Friedman, M. J. (1982). *Preventive mental health services for children entering foster home care.* White Plains, NY: Center for Preventive Psychiatry.

Kluft, R. P. (1986). Treating children who have multiple personality disorder. In B. G. Braun (Ed.), *Treatment of multiple personality disorder.* Washington, DC: American Psychiatric Press.

Kraus, M. (1971). Predicting success of foster placement for school aged children. *Social Work, 16,* 62–72.

Leon, E. (1979). *Running the first mile successfully.* Sacramento: Leon, Leon, Leon.

Littner, N. (1980). *More.* New York: Child Welfare League of America.

Maluccio, A. N., & Fein, E. (1983). Permanency planning: A redefinition. Child Welfare, *62,* 195–201.

Maluccio, A. N., & Sinanoglu, P. A. (Eds.). (1981). *The challenge of partnership: Working with parents of children in foster care.* New York: Child Welfare League of America.

Metropolitan Court Judges Committee. (1986). *Deprived children: A judicial response, 73 recommendations.* Reno: National Council of Juvenile and Family Court Judges.

Murray, J. P. (1983). *Status offenders: A source book.* Boys Town, NE: Boys Town Center.

National Commission on Children in Need of Parents. (1979). *Who knows? Who Cares? Forgotten children in foster care.* New York: Institute of Public Affairs.

Ordway, D. P. (1985). Standards for judicial determination in child maltreatment cases: A legal dilemma. In J. J. Cox & R. D. Cox (Eds.), *Foster care: Current issues, policies and practices.* Norwood, NJ: Ablex.

Pike, V., Downs, S., Emlen, A., Downs, G., & Case, D. (1977). *Permanency planning for children in foster care: A handbook for social workers* (DHEW publication 77-30124). Washington, DC: U.S. Department of Health, Education and Welfare.

Rutter, B. A. (1978). *The parents guide to foster family care.* New York: Child Welfare League of America.

Rutter, M. (1971). Parent-child separation: Psychological effects on the children. *Journal of Child Psychology and Psychiatry, 12,* 233–260.

Shyne, A. W., & Schroeder, A. G. (1978). *National study of social services to children and their families*. Washington, DC: Childrens Bureau for Children, Youth and Families, DHEW.

Sinanoglu, P. A., & Maluccio, A. N. (Eds). (1981). *Parents of children in placement: Prospectives and programs*. New York: Child Welfare League of America.

Sprouse, J. R. (1984). *Getting together: Organizing foster parent associations and support groups*. King George, VA: American Foster Care Resources.

Stack, C. B. (1985). Professional wisdom, cultural realities: Cross cultural perspectives on child welfare. In J. J. Cox & R. D. Cox (Eds.), *Foster care: Current issues, policies and practices*. Norwood, NJ: Ablex.

Swire, M. R., & Kavaler, F. (1977). The health status of foster children. *Child Welfare, 56*, 635–653.

Triseliotis, J. (1980). *New developments in foster and adoptive care*. London: Routlege and Kegan Paul.

Van Der Kolk, B. A. (1987). *Psychological trauma*. Washington, DC: American Psychiatric Press.

Vinokur-Kaplan, D., & Hartman, A. (1986). A national profile of child welfare workers and supervisors. *Child Welfare, 65*, 323–334.

PART II

Families of Adoption

Chapter 4

Adoption: Coping Constructively with the Social and Psychological Contexts

LOUISA ROGOFF-THOMPSON AND
JAMES W. THOMPSON

CHANGES IN ADOPTION: SOCIAL CONTEXT

THE DEMOGRAPHIC CONTEXT. Adoption has become a focus of growing public attention in the 1980s, reflecting a number of major demographic and attitudinal changes in the adopting parents, the children who are adopted, and the birth mothers who release them for adoption. People who adopt children today tend to be older than in the past. One reason for this is that many members of the baby-boom generation delayed starting their families until they entered the years of declining fertility. For many infertile couples, adoption becomes the most promising method of creating a family. Single people wishing to become parents also are turning to adoption. They, too, are usually older, having waited some years before concluding that they would not marry. Some couples who already have one or more children adopt older children because of a belief in zero population growth, or for health or other reasons.

There also have been changes in the demographic profile of "waiting children," i.e., children awaiting release for adoption. As in the past, many are the children of unwed mothers, and others have been removed from the custody of neglectful or abusive parents. Nowadays, greater acceptance of handicapped people in the mainstream of American life, combined with a decline in institutions to care for them, has

LOUISA ROGOFF-THOMPSON • Suburban Mental Health Associates, Baltimore, Maryland 21228.   JAMES W. THOMPSON • Department of Psychiatry, University of Maryland School of Medicine, Baltimore, Maryland 21201.

vastly increased the number of "special needs" adoptions. Indeed, because of de-institutionalization (the replacement of orphanages by foster care and adoption), many adoption agencies now devote almost all their time to special needs adoptions.

News of refugee children in Southeast Asia and, more recently, El Salvador, has inspired adoption for humanitarian reasons. There also is a tradition of adoption of mixed-race children of American servicemen, from Korea and Southeast Asia. India and some Latin American countries have permitted Americans to adopt children from their orphanages and hospitals, and some agencies have come to specialize in these foreign adoptions.

The age at which children are adopted has changed, too. In the early and mid-20th century, babies were quite often adopted at or shortly after birth. Today there is less stigma attached to raising a child out of wedlock, and many unwed mothers do so, at least for a few months or years. Then, if they find they cannot adequately care for their children, they may release them for adoption. Sometimes parents involuntarily lose custody of their children, who are then placed in foster care until they can return home or until released for adoption. Thus, many of the children waiting for adoption are school-aged, and even adolescent.

Those women who do give their babies up at birth seem to turn away from adoption agencies. This is so pervasive a phenomenon in regard to white babies that many agencies today routinely answer inquiries with a statement that they place almost no healthy white babies. Agency adoptions are now largely confined to placement of older, foreign, and minority group children, as well as children of all races who have special needs. In the past, many of these children have been reared in orphanages or by relatives.

Nonetheless, it should be emphasized that one can still adopt a healthy white newborn. White babies are being adopted in considerable numbers, through a variety of independent (formerly referred to as "private") adoption processes. Independent adoption involves direct placement of the baby by the birth mother, with or without the help of an intermediary such as a physician or attorney. Independent adoption, regulated by many states and by an Interstate Compact on the Placement of Children,* is not more expensive than agency adoption. Usually, the adopting couple pays the birth mother's uninsured medical

---

*The Interstate Compact on the Placement of Children is a uniform law that has been enacted by almost all states. It establishes orderly procedures for the interstate placement (adoption or foster care) of children and fixes responsibility for those involved in placing the child. See the *Guide to the Interstate Compact on the Placement of Children,* published by the American Public Welfare Society (Washington, D.C, 1981) for an explanation of the compact, and the uniform text of the laws.

expenses, her attorney (if she wants one), and their own attorney. States that regulate independent adoption normally do not permit the attorneys or other intermediaries to charge more than their customary hourly rates for the work they do.

Black market (illegal) and "gray market" (questionably legal) adoptions have received considerable publicity but probably are not very common. In a black market adoption, the birth mother sells her child; i.e., she receives compensation beyond her medical and legal expenses. The intermediary who locates the child may receive very high fees. It is clearly illegal to buy a child (under the antislavery laws), but (depending on the particular state's laws) it is not necessarily illegal to pay high fees to the intermediary. The term *gray market*, though sometimes used pejoratively to refer to any nonagency adoption, is most appropriately used when the adoption is not illegal, but some exploitation is involved, such as very high intermediary's fees.

THE FAMILY AND ETHNIC CONTEXT. Where once the birth mother, an agency, a judge, and the adopting couple were the sole parties involved in making placement decisions, now rights have been granted to a number of other individuals and groups. In many states, the birth father, if known, must be sought out and, if located after a reasonable search, must give his consent to the adoption before it can take place. The birth father or his relatives may choose to raise the baby, even if the birth mother prefers to place the baby elsewhere.

In the past, as today in foreign adoptions, it was possible (particularly for a white couple) to adopt a child of a different race or ethnic group. Today, in domestic adoptions, there are often agency regulations and state and federal laws restricting this. By federal act (the Indian Child Welfare Act of 1978),* if a baby has American Indian ancestry, the tribe must be involved in the placement of the baby, with priority given to adoption by Indian parents. This is an attempt to correct the previous practice of removing children from the tribes and placing them with white couples (in an ideologically motivated attempt to force Indians to become assimilated into white society). The Indian Child Welfare Act also explicitly states the policy that it is better for the child to be raised by members of his or her own ethnic group than to be adopted cross-culturally.

Similarly, many states will not permit a white couple to adopt an Afro-American child, or vice versa, presumably because of a belief that the child's psychological identity would suffer; in this case, the rights of an ethnic community are implied, and its preference assumed, without any specific consultation required from any individual or group. There

*Indian Child Welfare Act of 1978 (Public Law 95-608, 25 U.S.C.A., 1901–1963 (Supp. 1979).

have been cases in which white couples were refused the right to adopt Afro-American children even though no other parents could be found for them because they were handicapped or otherwise hard to place.

Foreign adoptions are often interracial and almost always transcultural. Perhaps this is why many countries refuse to allow their children to be adopted into other countries. In the United States, because of widespread recognition of the need to preserve the child's ethnic identity and cultural heritage, parents and agencies involved in foreign adoptions have created groups like the Latin American Parents Association (LAPA),* Families Adopting Children Everywhere (FACE),† and Organization for a United Response (OURS).‡ These groups offer parents help in maintaining their children's dual identities as, for example, American and Hispanic, Korean, or Indian. Their national and local newsletters publish personal accounts of families coping with cross-cultural adjustments, and contain everything from ethnic recipes to accounts of visits to various countries and information about medical and social problems common to children adopted from foreign countries. They also serve as a clearinghouse for information about local groups and events of interest. Their local chapters offer the children a peer group with similar ethnic heritages, and serve as a support group for the parents.

A general resource on adoption groups is the North American Council on Adoptable Children (NACAC),§ which publishes several helpful information booklets. NACAC is a union of citizen groups concerned with adoption. Like the other organizations mentioned above, it is not an adoption agency and does not place children.

Another change in the social context of adoption, particularly in domestic adoptions, is increasing openness. The last two decades have seen the publications of many stories by adopted children of their search for their birth parents (among the earliest and most influential were

---

*Latin American Parents Association (LAPA), P.O. Box 72, Seaford, New York 11783. LAPA publishes a national newsletter and has local chapters.

†Families Adopting Children Everywhere (FACE) is one of many local and regional organizations devoted to providing support for adoptive parents and their children. (FACE specializes in Asian children.) Its address is P.O. Box 28058, Northwood Station, Baltimore, Maryland 21239.

‡Organization for a United Response (OURS) is an umbrella organization for such groups as FACE, oriented toward international adoption. It is a good resource to locate such an organization in a given area of the country. It can be reached at OURS, Inc., 3307 Highway 100 North, Suite 203, Minneapolis, Minnesota 55422. OURS publishes a national magazine.

§North American Council on Adoptable Children, Inc., 1346 Connecticut Avenue, N.W., Suite 229, Washington, D.C. 20036. NACAC publishes the *Adoption Help Directory,* the *Directory of Adoptive Parent Groups,* and a newsletter. The organization also has other print and video materials on adoption, and has coordinators in every state.

Fisher, 1973; Lifton, 1975, 1979; Lowry, 1978), and this has fueled a move toward more open adoptions. A generation or two ago, when children could be raised without knowing that they were adopted, the identity of the adopting parents was protected, too, so that the birth parents could not later reclaim the child. Today, adoption agencies typically permit and often encourage some exchange of information, while independent adoptions range from completely anonymous to completely open—i.e., with ongoing contact between the birth parent(s) and the child.

Although this latter form of adoption, in which the child grows up knowing two sets of parents, has received some publicity lately, in independent adoptions it is more common for birth parents and adopting parents to meet in public places, use first names only, and exchange minimal identifying information. The birth mother may supply information about herself and the child's other birth relatives to be made available to the child at a later date; this may include identifying information (to enable the child to locate her), medical records, and more personal information such as photographs and letters. She may also request that photographs be sent to her periodically, directly, or through her lawyer.

Thus, demographic and attitudinal changes have created many new options for birth parents, for adopting parents, and for children who in the past might not have been adopted into American homes. All of these changes bring new challenges, some of them very difficult ones. Yet we will argue that the greatest challenges are those that have always been part of adoption: resolving one's grief over the losses entailed. For each person involved in an adoption, this is an issue that must be dealt with, lest the unhealed grief lead to future difficulties. In the following sections, we focus on the losses that surround or precede an adoption. In the final section, we will discuss the need for resolution of one's feelings about these losses, in order to handle the successive challenges of adoption more effectively.

THE PSYCHOLOGICAL CONTEXT OF ADOPTION

Loss. Loss is an important fact for almost everyone involved in adoption. The birth mother loses her child. Neufeld (1983) portrays the painful soul-searching that this can involve. Birth fathers, too, may go through this process (Eyerly, 1977). In addition, the release of the child for adoption also may be experienced as the loss of a family member by the birth mother's parents or relatives, and by any other children she has and is raising. In short, anyone who would have been part of the child's family if the child were not adopted may experience loss. While, nowadays, birth fathers often have the right to take part in the placement decision, most of these other family members do not. Even when members of the child's birth family have an opportunity to express their wishes, they may do so under pressure to make a decision fairly quickly. There is as yet little widespread understanding or systemic support for them.

In contrast to the birth relatives' experience of loss, the adopted child's loss is relatively well understood, or at least well publicized as a result of the many books and articles on the subject (in addition to the personal accounts listed above, see Sorosky, Baran, & Pannor, 1978). Some common themes are a sense of rejection and uncertainty about one's identity. Not every adopted child necessarily grows up with a sense of rejection and loss, but if other experiences create such feelings (as can happen to any child, adopted or not), the knowledge that one is adopted can come to symbolize and intensify them. Identity confusion too, can be intensified by a sense of alienation from one's roots, or a feeling of differentness from one's family, that can stem from adoption.

Infertility: Symbolic Loss. Adopting parents also suffer loss, two-fold and all too often unacknowledged: the loss of their own actual or potential birthchildren (whether miscarried, stillborn, dead in infancy, or never even conceived but vividly imagined), and the loss of a part of their identity as men and women. Even support groups such as RE-SOLVE* (a nationwide organization for people with infertility problems) tend to foster the belief that a successful adoption ends the sense of loss. Becoming a new parent is such an absorbing experience that there is little emotional energy left for grieving, yet the grief process may well be only dormant, to reawaken later.

Because infertility is the aspect of loss with which we, the authors, are personally familiar, we shall discuss it at length, hoping that this will also serve to provoke thought about the grief process for the other parties to adoption. We will present this discussion largely from the woman's point of view, since this volume is about women.

Infertility and Loss of the Dream Child. For a woman, the "dream child" is the child she has dreamed of having, the child she would carry in her body for 9 months, give birth to, and perhaps nurse. For both parents, the dream child is the child who would be a miracuous blend of the two of them, the child who would carry on their genes and cultural heritages.

For some couples, the dream child is the child who was conceived but then lost. (Some kinds of infertility involve failure to carry a child to term, so that couples experience repeated miscarriages or stillbirths.

---

*RESOLVE, Inc., is a national organization that is concerned with infertility. It has a national newsletter and many local chapters. The main office is RESOLVE, Inc., 5 Water Street, Arlington, Massachusetts 02174.

Parents who lose a child through the sudden infant death syndrome and genetic diseases that cause death in infancy also experience this loss.) The loss of a child through miscarriage, stillbirth, or infant death, can be shattering. (Panuthos & Romeo, 1984, offer an excellent discussion of the experience of childbearing loss, and of means of recovery from it.) Some bereaved parents try to avoid experiencing their grief by focusing on the future, immediately trying to become pregnant again or to adopt, and possibly subjecting themselves to another loss or disappointment. On the other hand, loss of a child or even a pregnancy often provides a sufficient context for mourning, so that the parents can allow themselves time to go through the entire grief process.

For other infertile couples, the dream child was present only in fantasy, so there is no tangible focus for grief. The couple who cannot conceive at all may have difficulty recognizing their grief for what it is. Both the treatment of infertility and the adoption process are fraught with uncertainty and frustration. Unrecognized feelings of grief can easily be transformed into feelings of anger, even outrage, toward unresponsive institutions (insurance companies, adoption agencies, and courts) and insensitive medical professionals.

For example, an infertile couple may find themselves ready to throttle a physician who casually informs them that it is time to start exploring the possibility of adoption. What is for the physician a matter of weighing probabilities and adding options can be, for the couple, a devastating indication of defeat that threatens their identities as individuals and as a couple.

Family members, still asking, "When are you going to have a baby?" also may elicit seemingly irrational feelings of anger, guilt, and failure. Almost all people with fertility problems delay telling their parents and siblings, in part because of a reluctance to admit to themselves that there is a problem, but also in part out of fear of condemnation, intrusiveness, and all the other inappropriate reactions that family members so often inflict on one another. Yet such a delay further removes one potential source of emotional support.

Sadly, as speakers at RESOLVE meetings repeatedly point out, spouses are sometimes not very helpful to one another, either, in dealing with infertility. This is in part because men and women tend to have different coping styles, but also because the losses involved are different for men and women. Clinical experience suggests that, while both may grieve for the dream child, the woman, more than the man, grieves for a lost part of her identity.

Infertility and Loss of Identity. What makes a woman a woman? For most of human history, motherhood was the central, essential core of womanhood. Yet, in recent decades, women have not been defined solely as wives and mothers. They have tried to distinguish womanhood from personhood—i.e., to delineate and strive to attain the qualities that make a good person, regardless of gender. For many women, professional identity has become the core of personal identity. Thoughts about motherhood, instead of taking precedence in identity formation, were often deferred or discounted. And yet, forgotten, discounted, or simply deferred, motherhood can assume much greater importance after other goals are met and other identities established, and still greater importance when it is threatened.

The same years that witnessed the broadening of women's identity also brought renewed interest in natural childbirth, breastfeeding, day care, and early childhood education, and the means by which a working mother can be a good mother. Many women discuss, read, and think about all of these subjects extensively, long before they ever try to become pregnant. Such conversations, readings, and fantasies all contribute to the formation of an identity as a future mother. Infertility threatens this identity on many levels.

Some women wish not to have children. Some do not find the "right" husband and thus experience a broader sense of loss and a different threat to their identity as women than comes from infertility. But many come to a point in their lives when they are ready and eager to have children. The frustration of that desire leads to a host of unexpected questions, accusations, and despairing thoughts: Can one be a complete woman yet not be fertile? . . . What were all those years of menstruation (and cramps) for? . . . My body doesn't work right; I feel like a cripple, an amputee. . . . Am I now less sexual, less attractive? . . . Part of me is dead. . . . Maybe I wasn't meant to be a mother. . . . What did I do to deserve this? Maybe I'm being punished for that abortion I had in college. . . . Maybe I brought this on myself by using the pill or the IUD, or by sleeping around and getting VD. . . .

Some of these thoughts are common; some just examples of the ideas that occur to each individual infertile woman, depending on the personal experiences.

Sexuality and reproduction may be experienced as quite separate when one is practicing contraception, but they merge when one is trying to become pregnant. Difficulties related to sexuality seem to be almost universal concerns addressed at RESOLVE meetings. There are external reasons for this: Infertility treatment involves a massive change in the sexual relationship. Coitus must occur at certain times of the month, and preferably not for a day or two before those presumed fertile days. Postcoital tests follow. The man gives semen samples. The woman submits to a number of painful and intrusive diagnostic procedures. Artificial insemination of her husband's or a donor's semen may be tried, accentuating the mechanistic aspects of what was once a joyful, loving act. In vitro fertilization takes this approach even further. Because these procedures are usually repeated once a month for several months, before giving way to the next procedure, years may go by during which the couple's sexual relationship not only has a forced quality but is associated with repeated failure. In this context, spontaneity is lost and, with it, a belief in one's sexual desirability.

RESPONSES TO LOSS

Maladaptive Responses: Avoidance of Grieving. Disappointment and a sense of loss easily lead to feelings of guilt or anger; one looks for someone or something to blame. Blame can be talked about more easily than loss, particularly losses in identity, because blame suggests fault and actions. At the least, it allows one to focus on past actions and produces a straightforward emotional response of guilt or anger. Sometimes the marriage flounders because of the need to blame someone; some couples choose an external target for their anger (Kraft et al., 1980).

Constructive coping mechanisms, too, can mask and delay dealing with loss. With doctors, family members including the spouse, friends, and even professionals who try to offer support, the first question is apt to be: What is wrong and what can be done about it? And because these discussions can be very extensive indeed (the medical aspects of infertility can be extraordinarily complex, the treatment a matter of months or years, and productive of another whole host of feelings that need to be expressed), it often happens that no one addresses the more threatening questions of identity and loss.

When the medical options (or the couple's patience with them) run out, adoption may be seen as the solution, the end of all this agonizing uncertainty, this disruptive treatment, this frustration about not being a parent yet. Adoption does offer a solution to many of these problems, yet there is another period of uncertainty, frustration, and (usually) new disappointments during the waiting period, until one day the child arrives. The new mother (and father) begins to experience a series of events out of which a new identity will emerge. Unfortunately, that new identity is not necessarily congruent with the one constructed in fantasy and expectations during all the years of wanting to have a child.

A woman learns how to be a mother, in part, by being one, but she also has had a lifetime of learning about how to be a mother, based primarily on her observation of her own mother, and her knowledge and feelings about that relationship. That relationship was between two people who shared a body for 9 months and then spent many years exploring their shared genetic heritage. A new mother looking at her adopted child does not see reflections of her own face, or her husband's, or her family's.

In time she will see reflections of her values and teachings, and of shared memories and experiences, but in the meanwhile, her child will demonstrate many unfamiliar gifts and equally unfamiliar difficulties. Thus, there may be an exceptionally wide disparity between the dream child and the adopted child, and, in turn, a lack of integration between the mother-I-am-becoming and the mother-I-thought-I-would-be.*

The degree to which this is so depends, in part, on how different the child is from the child one anticipated, but it also depends on the degree to which the woman has resolved her ambivalence about the adoption and the problems that led to it. Unfinished mourning for the dream child, or damage to a woman's identity, can make it difficult for a woman to accept her adopted child as "my" child, and can change parenthood from a state of being to an artificial role being played. This is true even though parents wholeheartedly love the child. The unexpected paradox, so rarely discussed by adoption workers or support groups, is that loving a child does not automatically produce a feeling that the child is your son or daughter. The unhealed emotional wounds left over from the experience of infertility may stand in the way.

The adoption of a child brings a new source of self-esteem that can help to replace or replenish the lost one, but it also brings new demands on time and energy. Couples who give birth to a child often experience a diminution of their sexual relationship in the months following the birth process, because of sheer fatigue. Adopting couples, too, are tired and have less time for each other. This reinforces the difficulty in restoring the sexual relationship, and it becomes a new reason to avoid dealing with that underlying identity problem: Am I truly a woman? Am I a sexual person? How can anyone be attracted to this inadequate part of me?

One of the most difficult aspects of this identity problem is that it is not usually shared. RESOLVE counselors have found that couples tend not to go through the infertility experience in a mutually supportive way. Infertility means different things to different men and women, and elicits different coping mechanisms. Even men who love children and long to be fathers, and who feel an emptiness in their lives when they do not have children, are less likely to have grown up with future fatherhood as a significant part of their identity. They are more likely to turn to action as their sole or primary way of dealing with infertility, and they may be baffled by a woman's need to explore the emotional aspects. In turn, her husband's lack of understanding of her identity conflicts, or his rejection of grieving as a healthy way of coping, leaves the

---

*This, and other ideas in this chapter, were derived from conversations with Susan G. Mikesell, Ph.D., a clinical psychologist practicing in Washington, D.C., who has treated many infertile couples. We gratefully acknowledge Dr. Mikesell's contributions to our thinking on the subject.

woman feeling more uncertain of herself, more defective, and more alienated.

Resolution of Grief and Building a New Identity. Given time and support from other family members or from professionals experienced in this field, a woman can build a new identity. The near-universal need of infertile women is to find someone who understands. In every RE-SOLVE support group and in every issue of its newsletters, women express their relief at having found, at last, people who have shared the same experience. Bringing the feelings out into the open, talking about them with people who can empathize, enables the woman to resolve her grief fully. Then the healing process can begin.

Once this shift from grieving to healing has occurred, the experience of motherhood through adoption offers a woman new, positive elements to be integrated into her identity, and new sources of self-esteem and self-knowledge. It offers a new arena for relating to her husband, so that even if the old relationship seems gone for good, a new one can grow.

Similarly, the birth mother, if she can complete a healthy griefwork for her lost child, can come to terms with her feelings about giving up her baby. Instead of seeing herself in negative terms primarily, she can focus on herself as a woman who did the best thing for her baby, an adult who could make a sacrifice when needed, an adult who could assess a situation realistically and understand that no solution is perfect but an adequate one can be found, a woman who has taken a responsible action, who has learned from experience, and who may be more responsible in the future. One day she may be ready to be a mother, and can build an identity as a mother on that earlier identity.

CONSTRUCTIVE DECISION MAKING AND PSYCHOLOGICAL GROWTH

A woman who releases her child for adoption makes a very difficult decision. She may make it impulsively, when her child is born, or she may think about it for months before or after the birth. Even if she makes it quickly, she must convince a judge that she has thought it through. If she begins early in her pregnancy to plan for her as yet unborn child, she can choose an agency that will give her a voice in selecting the adopting parents. Alternatively, she can choose the parents herself, in an independent adoption process. Thus, there is a good deal she can do to shape her child's future life, if she wants to take an active role. In turn, her actions on her child's behalf can help restore her self-esteem.

The adopting parents go through a more complicated process involving a sequence of decisions. They must first decide that they want to adopt. This does not necessarily imply a decision to stop trying to become pregnant, but in practice, it frequently means an end to medical interventions. There is a grieving process over the loss of the genetic child, as well as pregnancy, birth, and breastfeeding. The decision is made that it is more important to become parents now than to pursue those other goals.

This decision is only the beginning, however. The next step is to find out how to adopt. Initial inquiries often lead to considerable discouragement. If the couple is white, most agencies inform them that they cannot expect to adopt a newborn, or even an older white baby. Many agencies have waiting lists several years long, and they also may screen out potential parents according to a host of criteria such as age, health, and whether the woman works. Sometimes these criteria seem quite arbitrary, more designed to decrease the number of applicants rather than to select good parents.

If the couple persists, they learn about foreign, "special needs," and independent adoption. Independent adoption offers the hope of finding a healthy baby but transfers to the couple all of the uncertainties and responsibilities that any agency would have handled for them. They must find a birth mother who wants to surrender her baby, and risk the possibility that she will change her mind when the baby is born. This happens often; most of the couples of our acquaintances who have adopted this way have had at least one adoption fall through. This loss can be excruciating for people who have already suffered through years of infertility, and some change their minds and turn to other options.

There is room for negotiations between birth mother and adopting parents in independent adoption. If the baby has not yet been born, there are decisions and commitments to be made about the degree of openness versus anonymity of both parties, prenatal care, choice of hospital, whether the adopting parents can be present at the birth, and whether the birth mother will smoke, drink, or use drugs during her pregnancy. The adopting parents want the birth mother to provide the ideal prenatal environment for their baby, but they also do not want to annoy the birth mother to such an extent that she will reject them. However, in the experience of a number of adoption attorneys and adoptive parents, when an independent adoption occurs, there tends to be a rapid consensus in all these areas. It is when the birth mother or the adopting couple harbor doubts about whether they really want to go through with the adoption per se that they are likely to stall the negotiations.

For many people, the uncertainties involved in independent adoption are too stressful. Uncertainty is a central feature of the experience of infertility, and the desire to end it may be a motivating factor in the decision to adopt, so it is natural to wish to avoid it in the adoption process. Even agency adoptions involve uncertainty, but there is a greater sense of certainty that one day a child will arrive, and there are fewer decisions to be made by the couple. The trade-off is that an agency-placed child will rarely be a healthy newborn of the couple's own ethnic background.

One adoption worker said to us, "We want you to see how far you can 'stretch.'" She meant: What challenges could we take on that we had never even thought about before? Could we adopt a mentally retarded child, or one with a physically or emotionally handicapping condition, or one who would need surgery or extensive treatment of some other kind? Every couple expecting a baby has fears that these tragedies will occur, but it is quite different to choose one of them voluntarily. Some people who already have children feel confident enough to take on this more difficult parenting experience. Sometimes, people who are not acceptable candidates to agencies who place infants—because they are single or handicapped, for instance—turn to special needs adoption with varying degrees of misgiving. Some couples who decide to adopt realize that they have grown enough through the experience of infertility to help a child deal with similar experiences of doctors, disappointments, stigma, and so on.

In regard to special needs adoption, it is important to be aware that the initial barrage of information about severely handicapped children is intended to test how far the adoptive parents can "stretch." Later on, the adoption workers may reveal that there are other hard-to-place children who are not so handicapped or have visual impairment. To many of us, that seems quite normal, not a reason to reject a child. They may have siblings who need to be adopted along with them—and that could seem like a wonderful gift, not a handicap at all. The goal is to fit the child's needs to the parents' capabilities. To one couple, a learning disability may be a tragedy, while to another, it is a familiar fact of life.

It also happens that the experience of learning about specific children, with their minor and major problems, can make the children so real that the potential parent can envision raising *that* child, can begin to figure out how she or he would deal with *that* problem, and can see this as just part of parenting. The prospective parent grows and takes the problem in stride.

We have said that adoption begins with loss, and that each person's resolution of the grief over those losses is essential if the adoption is to be a success. For adults, ideally, this should occur before the adoption, but often there is so much else going on that grieving is deferred. Sometimes, by taking responsible action on behalf of the child—i.e., by acting like good parents—birth parents and adopting parents build up their self-esteem and emotional strength sufficiently enough to allow them to face the difficult challenges to their identity left over from the experience that led them to adoption. For the adopting parents, the loving relationship with the new child also contributes to, even if it does not ensure, resolution of grief.

For the adopted child, knowledge of their loss may not come until later. In today's context of greater openness about adoption, both sets of parents (birth and adoptive) may have the opportunity to help the child come to terms with the loss. For this reason, it is all the more important for each adult to have come to a healthy resolution of the conflicts involved.

We hope we have conveyed that, if the context of adoption always includes loss, it also offers an avenue to growth. Above all, we believe that attempts to dismiss or minimize the pain necessarily shut off the healing process, and the unhealed emotional wounds impair one's ability to love. As a wound should bleed freely and then be exposed to air, these feelings too should be released in a healing environment of empathic listeners. Only then can the shift occur, from using energy to contain the grief, to using it for growth and love.

REFERENCES

Eyerly, J. (1977). *He's my baby, now.* New York: Pocket Books.
Fisher, F. (1973). *The search for Anna Fisher.* Greenwich, CT: Fawcett Books.
Kraft, A. D., Palombo, J., Mitchell, D., Dean, C., Meyers, S., & Schmidt, A. W. (1980). The psychological dimensions of infertility. *American Journal of Orthopsychiatry, 50*(4), 618–628.
Lifton, B. J. (1975). *Twice born: Memoirs of an adopted daughter.* New York: McGraw-Hill.
Lifton, B. J. (1979). *Lost and found: The adoption experience.* New York: Dial Press.
Lowry, L. (1978). *Find a stranger, say good-bye.* Boston: Houghton Mifflin.
Neufeld, J. (1983). *Sharelle.* New York: Signet.
Panuthos, C., & Romeo, C. (1984). *Ended beginnings: Healing childbearing losses.* New York: Warner Books.
Sorosky, A. D., Baran, A., & Pannor, R. (1978). *The adoption triangle: The effects of the sealed record on adoptees, birth parents, and adoptive parents.* New York: Anchor Press/Doubleday.

Chapter 5

Adopting Children from Other Cultures

S. Peter Kim

The adoption of children from other cultures can be divided into two categories: the adoption of children who were born in a foreign country of dissimilar culture (international transcultural adoption), and the adoption of racially different children who were born in the same country as the adoptive parents and whose ethnic group maintains a distinctive identity within the parents' social framework (domestic transcultural adoption). In the cases of international adoption, the majority of the adopted children are racially different from the adoptive parents. Therefore, I have used the term *transcultural adoption* to imply transracial adoption.

History of Adoption in the United States

The purpose, concepts, and patterns of adoption have changed considerably in the United States during the past 50 years and continue to be in a process of change. In the early 16th century, Spanish immigrants brought to the United States the influence of Roman adoption, which almost exclusively served the needs of the adopter (Huard, 1956; Presser, 1971). Over the years, however, the basic purpose of adoption changed to benefit primarily children who needed homes. More children are legally adopted in this country than in the rest of the world as a whole (Baran, Sorosky, & Pannor, 1975). The interest in adoption is not confined to childless couples, and a growing number of fertile couples are seeking to become adoptive parents (Joe, 1978). Single-parent adop-

S. Peter Kim • Medical College of Georgia, Augusta, Georgia 30912.

tion by those who never were married or are divorced has emerged as a new trend in the last decade of this country.

In the late 1930s, there were many children waiting for adoption, but there were not many available homes. The adopting family had to go to great lengths to find a perfect infant, one who would most closely match their physical characteristics. The insistence on physical matching was reinforced, if not initiated, by adoption agencies. Every effort was made to match ethnic background, skin color, and intellectual potential. When the economy improved after World War II, more white couples wanted to adopt children, and the supply of white infants decreased. Adoption requirements then shifted to emphasize the "perfect" adoptive homes, which could be provided almost exclusively by white parents, who were legally married, religiously devout, respected in the community, and prosperous, but childless. Thus, the adoption stereotype became entrenched in the image of the "perfect" baby going to the "perfect" home (Feiertag, 1973).

The factors of religion, race, and social class often were used to exclude prospective parents and/or adoptees from the process. A review of transracial adoption in the United States suggests that the beginning of such procedures was by happenstance. Before the mid-1950s, the absence of official policies about transracial adoptions did not prohibit such placements. Most, if not all, of the first transracial adoptions were implemented through highly personalized procedures (Ladner, 1978).

In the mid-1950s and thereafter, the widespread use of contraceptive measures, liberalized abortion laws, and the increased number of white mothers who decided to keep their out-of-wedlock infants further diminished the supply of adoptable white babies. At the same time there was a rapid increase in children who were "hard to place"—those who were nonwhite, beyond infancy, and physically and emotionally handicapped. By far the greatest number of these hard-to-place children were nonwhite. (A nonwhite child is defined by most adoption agencies as one who is known not to have two Caucasian biological parents; the category includes blacks, Hispanics, American Indians, and Asians.) Despite efforts by various adoption agencies, the number of adoptable nonwhite children continued to increase. These children are conservatively estimated to number 50,000 (United States Department of Health, Education and Welfare, 1976).

In the United States the adoption of children from foreign countries, mainly from Sweden and Japan, began in the mid-1940s, although the war-orphaned children brought to America were insignificant in number. Since the early 1950s, with conflicts in Korea and Vietnam, a large number of Asian children have been brought into the United States for adoption by middle- and upper-middle-class white families.

American adoption agencies began a concerted effort to place black children who were in need of adoption (Chestang, 1972; Falk, 1970; Gallay, 1963; Lebo, Rogers, & Stuhlmann, 1965; Madison & Schapiro, 1973). This effort intensified after publications of the National Adoption Survey of the Child Welfare League of America and the National Conference of Adoption in 1955 (Chestang, 1972) reported that an increasingly large number of black children remained to be adopted.

The Children's Service Center of Montreal pioneered transracial adoption placement beginning in 1958. The Open Door Society, possibly the first autonomous adoptive parents' organization, was chartered in Montreal in 1962 by three families who had adopted children across racial lines (Madison & Schapiro, 1973). One of the society's objectives was to stimulate adoption agencies to find and encourage white applicants to adopt nonwhite children. Similar developments occurred in the United States, and Open Door Societies have been instituted in many American cities.

Although recent accurate figures are not available, the number of foreign adoptions increased by more than three times between 1968 and 1975, from 1,612 to 5,633 (United States Immigration and Naturalization Service, 1968–1975). However, the overall rate for adoptions declined (Joe, 1978). Of 27,242 children placed for adoption by agencies in this country in 1974, 4,770 were international adoptions, and 3,813 were placements of black children (Boys and Girls Aid Society, 1976; Cole, 1976). Actually, the number of black children adopted has declined moderately.

Only one-third or one-quarter of black children waiting for adoption are adopted by white families, while almost all the foreign adoption placements are in white families (Madison & Schapiro, 1973). Projections of these data suggest that the issues of the transcultural and transracial adoptions cannot be regarded as on the periphery of adoption in this country. Yet little is known about the developmental and sociological impact of the recent trends of increasing international adoption and decreasing or sedentary adoption of black children on the involved children, adoptive families, and American adoption practice in general. More studies need to be directed toward this area.

ADOPTIVE FAMILIES

Several studies have focused on the psychosocial aspects of the transracially adopting parents and their families (Falk, 1970; Fricke, 1965; Gallay, 1963; Ladner, 1978; Lebo et al., 1965). The findings of these studies generally suggest that transracially adopting couples tend to be at higher socioeconomic levels and adopt mostly out of religious and humanitarian motives when compared with couples adopting racially similar children, who more frequently state they adopted to have a child or another child. My colleagues and I (Kim, Hong, & Kim, 1979) conducted a study of 21 Korean children adopted by 15 white couples. Thirteen of these couples listed as their primary reason for adoption the desire to have a child or children; only 2 couples said their motive was to provide an orphan with a home.

Transracially adopting couples tend to be geographically or socially isolated from the members of their extended family and may rely on the social interaction and emotional support of friends. Childrearing tends to be a conscious and carefully planned experience for the adoptive parents (Ladner, 1978). They are more active in community and civic work than parents who adopt children of the same race. Although the transracially adopting couples experience very few difficulties with their community members because of the transracial adoption (Fricke, 1965), about two-fifths of the transracially adopted schoolchildren have experienced some difficulties because of race (Falk, 1970), such as hecklings from classmates or difficulties in making new friends. The transracially adopted children in rural regions, compared with large cities, tend to experience more difficulties.

More transracially adopting couples had borne children than had couples adopting children of the same race. The transracially adopting parents are more likely to report special publications and social agencies as first sources of information leading to adoption; parents who adopt within their race more frequently report pastors or friends as first sources.

Kirk (1964) has suggested that men are relatively more hesitant than women to accept adoption. In the initial decisions to investigate adoption, the transracially adopting husband played a larger role than the husband who adopted within his race. The transracially adopting wife played a lesser role than did the wife who adopted within her race, although the differences were not great among the wives (Falk, 1970).

There is little variance among all adoptive couples in how frequently they have felt hurt or disturbed by remarks about their adoptions. However, the transracially adopting couples report few incidents of harassment (Fricke, 1965).

White adoptive parents of biracial and/or black children have reported experiencing psychological hurt because of the adoption (Ladner, 1978). The parents of the adoptive mother and/or father have been known to reject the idea of the child; the adoption is viewed as a family tragedy. Other adoptive grandparents gradually have accepted the adoption. In her study of transracially adoptive families, Ladner (1978) was apprised of derogatory comments directed toward the adopted children by their peers and of the hostile stares of others in public places. In some families, especially in integrated neighborhoods, the presence of a black adopted child seems to foster positive relationships between the biological siblings and other black youngsters in the neighborhood.

A majority of transracially adoptive couples indicate that they believe it is more difficult to rear an adopted child of a race other than their own. They are less willing to recommend transracial adoption than intraracially adoptive couples are willing to recommend intraracial adoption (Ladner, 1978).

Single-parent adoptions are very small in number; no precise nationwide demographic and psychosocial data currently are available. I have had only three single-parent adoption cases in my study group in the past 8 years. The parental profiles of these three adoptions present some similarities and uniformities. All of them (two white mothers and one fair-skinned Hispanic father of Puerto Rican nativity) were in their early 30s at the time of adoption and had had histories of early deprivations: The two mothers lost both parents (both mothers) in their early childhood; the father had been adopted by a same-ethnic family. Each adopted a black child of relatively "old age" (4-, 6-, and 7-year old boys). All three parents, college graduates, were in either managerial or professional occupations. One mother, a divorcee, had no children from her marriage and did not plan to remarry. The other two parents never had been married. They were not closed entirely to the idea, although they were aware of possible difficulties in finding spouses who would accept their adoptive children. None of the parents had maintained close ties with their respective families and appeared to be socially isolated.

The two mothers reported that they and their children had been harassed frequently by people they encountered; their children's conspicuously different appearance was seen as the reason. The Hispanic father and his son seldom had such experiences, perhaps because of the fairly close resemblance between himself and the child. In the presence of their adopted children, the mothers were often mistaken as social workers or temporary caretakers. Expressions of sympathy and/or admiration were offered; more often, comments were of a derogatory or condescending nature. These parents were better prepared to handle such negative encounters. Whenever possible and appropriate, they responded in a firm and polite manner. These encounters always were followed by the parents' supportive and reassuring talks with the children. Their love for the children and their commitment to them was emphasized. However, in the setting of the study, each parent expressed varying degrees of concern and uncertainty about the possible adverse developmental effects of single parenting and raised questions about providing the role models of the missing opposite-gender parent.

They were unduly sensitive to deviations in their children's emotional or behavioral patterns and concerned that they might develop into behavioral or psychiatric problems. They always were quick to seek professional assistance for advice about any minute behavioral changes of their children.

The single-parent/biracial adoption is a relatively new pattern. The long-term outcomes of such adoptions need to be studied in preparation for the possibility of an increase in these trends in the future.

Controversy over International Adoption

Joe (1978) has summarized the most prevalent criticisms of international adoption as follows: Such adoptions exploit children from poor countries, irregular adoption procedures encourage a black market, and foreign children become an exported problem and a drain on American taxpayers. Critics feel that foreign children should be assisted to remain in their own countries. Thus, needy American children will not be bypassed in favor of foreign children who, when they grow up, may never be accepted here. From these somewhat unfounded objections, the central issue of international adoption emerges: Is it proper for a child to become a permanent member of a family with a different biological and cultural heritage? The perennial question of heredity versus environment is resurrected, and although race and nationality do not determine each other, the issues in transracial and international adoption develop because most foreign adoptees differ visibly from their adoptive parents in racial or ethnic background.

Joe's (1978) argument in defense of international adoption is firmly based on her conviction that all human beings share a craving for a sense of belonging, and the form of that belonging is not mandated by the accidental political boundaries of birth—that is, the national identity. This view also is supported by Shibutani and Kwan (1965), who, in their sociological treatise on ethnicity, point out that human beings throughout the world are fundamentally alike in their anatomical structure, in their ability to engage in reflective thought, and in sharing a pool of common sentiments. The basic differences between ethnic groups are cultural, and the norms serve as masks to cover the basic similarities.

Although dealing with relatively small numbers, empirical studies of transracial and transcultural adoptions reveal that the adopted children tend to take on the characteristics of their new families and may actually suffer less from feelings of inferiority than do minority children of similar racial or ethnic heritage living in this country with biological parents (Fanshel, 1972; Ferguson, 1969). Many families with foreign adopted children provide a link between nationalities by incorporating aspects of the child's original culture into their daily life and maintaining associations with the child's native peoples both here and abroad. Some of the examples are to expose the child to foods, dress, and toys of the child's original culture, and family participation in the cultural affairs, such as museum visits, movies, and plays, depicting the child's original culture.

Controversy over Transracial Adoption

Several factors have led to the advocacy and practice of transracial adoption of black children (Chimezie, 1975). Among these are the disproportionately large number of black children, the perception (Herzog, 1971; Sharrar, 1971) that black families are reluctant to adopt black children, and the belief (Herzog, 1971; Sharrar, 1971) that, to develop a healthy personality, a child needs to be raised in a family by his or her own or adoptive parents. Other reasons include the belief that children raised in institutions or foster homes develop behavior problems and often are maladjusted, and the rarely mentioned psychosocial need of white parents to adopt black children (Sharrar, 1971).

The Child Welfare League of America, although it always has stressed the desirability of placing children with families of the same racial or ethnic background, took a cautious position on transracial adoption by stating that physical resemblances of the adoptive parents, the child, or his or her natural parents, should not be a determining factor in the selection of a home (Child Welfare League of America, 1968). Essentially, this position implies that a child should not be deprived of a family because of the unavailability of a prospective adoptive family of the same race. The league, during the early 1960s, in cooperation with the Bureau of Indian Affairs, facilitated the placement of a number of American Indian children in white adoptive homes. The league also has encouraged agencies to consider placing black children in white homes, pending the recruitment of a sufficient number of black adoptive homes (Grow & Shapiro, 1974).

During the late 1960s and early 1970s, as the preservation and maintenance of cultural and racial identity were stressed increasingly by minority groups, transracial adoption came under strong criticism from many quarters. Jones (1972), as one of the strongest opponents of transracial adoption, openly questioned the white adoptive parents' ability to grasp the totality of the problem of being black in American society, no matter how deeply imbued they were with goodwill. He further questioned the white parents' ability to help the adopted black children create a black identity and advocated permanent foster care and small-group care within the black community as a better alternative to the placement of black children in white families.

The objections against raising a black child or a child of a different culture in a white family are not based on the doubts about the white parents' ability to meet the child's need for material necessities or loving care. The contention is based on the concern that the white family may not equip the adopted child with the necessary psychosocial tools to develop an appropriate identity and deal with the oppression of a racist society (Chimezie, 1975). The issues of racial awareness and self-identify of the transracially adopted children have been studied, but the results are inconclusive (Chestang, 1972; Falk, 1969; Ladner, 1978; Simon, 1974).

The earlier studies (Goodman, 1964; Moreland, 1969) reported that nonwhite adopted children preferred white dolls over dolls of their own skin color. Simon (1974) studied levels of racial awareness, racial preferences, and racial identities among nonwhite children (120 American black, 37 Korean, and 10 American Indian) and compared their attitudes with those of 109 white siblings who had been born into the adopted families. She found that black children reared in the special setting of multiracial families did not acquire ambivalence toward their own race and also that there were no significant differences in racial attitudes among the adopted children in the other ethnic categories studied.

The long-term effect of transracial and transcultural adoption on the personality development of the adoptees remains controversial. Identity formation has been the main issue. Chestang (1972) and Chimezie (1975) have contended that transracial adoption adversely affects the children's psychological development and leads to .dentity crises mainly because they have been deprived of their own ethnic cultural experience and lack skills to cope with racism. However, Johnson (1976) and Vieni (1975) have suggested that transracial adoption is more beneficial to the children than institutionalization.

Berlin (1978) has called our attention to the long-term as well as the immediate developmental needs of transracially adopted children. He emphasized the need to preserve cultural ties in the case of American Indian children and perhaps for all minority children placed outside of their tradition. Such cultural ties should help to minimize these children's suffering and estrangement during adolescence.

The Incidence of Behavioral Symptoms and Psychiatric Disorders

Although the 1946 Curtis Report (Care of Children Committee, 1946) claimed that most conventional intraracial adoptions could be considered socially successful, the majority of other clinical reports and statistical data (Berlin, 1978; Clothier, 1939; Frisk, 1964; Goodman, Silberstein, & Mandell, 1963; Johnson, 1976; McWhinnie, 1969; Peller, 1963; Schechter, Carlson, Simmons, & Work, 1964; Vieni, 1975) show a 15 to

30% incidence of adoptees in the psychiatric population, which far exceeds the 2% incidence in the general census (Weider, 1977). Currently, there are no comprehensive data regarding the incidence of psychiatric disorders among the transracially or transculturally adopted children.

Grow and Shapiro (1974) studied 125 black children adopted by white parents. The children's mean age was 9 years; their mean adoption period was more than 7 years. Grow and Shapiro (1974) reported that a relatively frequent pattern of neurotic symptoms (bedwetting, nightmares, restlessness) occurred more among children under 12, among boys, among children with mothers under 40, and among those children adopted by small families of less than four household members. The fact that the child did not match the parents' intellectual preferences also was associated with these symptoms. A pattern of relatively frequent physical symptoms (colds, headaches, tiredness) appeared more often among children over 10 years old and also was seen more frequently in children described by their parents as not obviously black by skin color.

Rathbun and colleagues (Rathbun, DiVirgilio & Waldfogel, 1958; Rathbun, McLaughlin, Bennett, & Garland, 1965) studied 38 foreign children brought to the United States for adoption. The authors reported on the children's initial reactions to the shock of being transplanted into their new American families and also on their later adjustments. The initial reaction symptoms in about four-fifths of the children were regarded as mild or moderate. The symptoms of the other 20% of the children were considered severe. Thirty-three children (17 Greek, 12 Asian, 3 Italian, and 1 American-Turkish) of the original 38 were reevaluated 5 years later when their ages ranged from 6 to 16. The adjustment of 10 children was considered problematic; 2 were rated clinically disturbed and in need of professional help, chiefly in reaction to the adoptive home situation. The 2 disturbed children were adopted at an early age and were in latency at the time of reevaluation. In some cases the children in the study were subjected to early deprivation and even to abuse before they were transplanted at a critical age of ego development. They continued to struggle with unresolved identity problems complicated by the approach of adolescence.

My colleagues and I (Kim et al., 1979) studied 21 Korean children who had been adopted by 15 white couples. Nine adoptive couples reported behavioral symptoms in 16 children for whom they had sought or considered seeking professional help at one time. Among the 9 children who had been adopted before age 3, temper tantrums and excessive and frequent crying were the most commonly reported symptoms. Every child in this group was reported to have had temper tantrums, whereas only one-third of the children adopted after age 3 were reported to have this symptom. Two-thirds of the children adopted before age 3 exhibited excessive and frequent crying. Five children in this group had the combined symptoms of temper tantrums and excessive and frequent crying.

In the group of 12 children adopted after age 3, 8 exhibited learning difficulty and 7 exhibited shyness and withdrawing behavior, which were the most common symptoms. In this group, 3 children had a combination of learning difficulty and depression, and 3 other children showed combined symptoms of withdrawal and learning difficulty. When the two groups were combined, the incidence of four major behavioral symptoms was as follows: temper tantrums (62%), shyness and withdrawing behavior (43%), excessive and frequent crying (38%), and learning difficulty (38%).

In regard to learning difficulty, at the time of the survey 7 of the 9 children adopted before age 3 were below first-grade age; 10 of the 12 children adopted after age 3 were in first or a higher grade. There were no significant differences between boys and girls in the incidence of behavior symptoms. All children in the study were reported to be in good physical health since adoption, and none was diagnosed as having minimal brain dysfunction or fine motor-perceptual dysfunction.

Only 1 child of the 16 who manifested symptoms required psychiatric intervention, suggesting that the behavioral symptoms among the majority of adopted children may be viewed as only intensified, transient features of adjustment to their new environment. Temper tantrums and excessive crying among the very young adopted children were vexing problems to the inexperienced adoptive parents. Some parents became apprehensive and suspected that the children might have psychopathology or brain damage. A few parents harbored this suspicion long after negative tests.

Learning difficulties in the group of children adopted after age 3 usually appeared to be related to the problems of English language acquisition and acculturation, as well as to the shock of transcultural transplantation. Their shyness and withdrawal may be viewed as depression equivalents, resulting from complex factors such as culturally instilled temperament, painful experience of parental privation or deprivation early in life, and stress arising from the adjustment to a totally new environment.

I (Kim, 1980) have reported three cases of transracially adopted Korean children, 22 to 30 months old, who manifested transient but severe behavioral symptoms that resembled childhood psychosis, raising the question of the applicability of conventional psychiatric diagnostic classification to these children. A more careful examination of the phenomenon might be conducted through a multidimensional approach designed to understand these children's developmental psychodynamics. The three major dimensions to consider correlatively are the transcultural and transracial nature of adoption, the adoptive parents and family, and the child's unique developmental needs. The adoptive parents' understanding of the culture-specific childrearing customs of the child's former society is of particular importance when assessing the child's development.

It is comforting to note that in one major study (Grow & Shapiro, 1974) on 125 transracially adopted black children, 77% were judged to represent successful adoptions. This success rate is typical of adoption studies, whether of conventional adoption of white infants by white families or unconventional adoption across racial or cultural lines. No comparable study regarding black children adopted by black families has yet been made available.

REMAINING QUESTIONS

Most studies of transracial and transcultural adoption are limited in scope, depth, and number of subjects. Thus, they leave unanswered several questions that require further longitudinal investigation. Among areas of investigation are the following:

- The long-term effects of early behavioral symptoms in relation to development of personality and psychopathology.
- The patterns of attachment exhibited by children adopted during and after the so-called critical period of the first 2 years of life.
- The numerous possible changes in the adoptive families' social and financial circumstances, parental/marital stability, the effect of the adopted parents' attitudes and upbringing on the children's adjustment, and the behavioral and psychosocial reaction of the adopted children to society's slowly changing concept of racism.
- The correlation between English language acquisition (rapidity, proficiency, and capacity to conceptualize) and adjustment to new environments among children from non-English-speaking countries who were adopted after the age of 6.
- The development of racial awareness and self-identity in relation to patterns of social adjustment and achievement during latency and adolescence.
- Methods of helping adopted children preserve ties with their country of origin or their ethnic group.

CONCLUSION

The results of the available studies represent only the beginning of our understanding of transracial and transcultural adoptions in this area. Although the findings are inconsistent and bar any premature conclusion, one basic theme emerges: Minority children may be viewed as developmentally vulnerable, and the children and their adoptive families are under stress. While the controversies over the advisability of transracial and transcultural adoption continue, we must face the reality that an ever-increasing number of ethnic minority children await adoption in permanent homes, and more prospective adoptive parents are turning to transracial and overseas adoption. It is time for professionals dealing with child mental health, education, and social welfare to recognize these recent adoption trends and respond to the service needs of adoptive children and adoptive families.

An adoption agency under the auspices of the Department of Health and Human Services or a voluntary agency with federal sponsorship should be established to oversee American adoption practices and research projects, especially transracial and transcultural adoption. Representatives of ethnic and cultural minorities should be included among the agency staff or advisory board experts in child mental health, education, and social services. The agency should establish basic guidelines and policies of adoption and supervise their implementation and also should serve as an information clearinghouse for private adoption agencies and the numerous self-help adoptive parents' organizations throughout the country. The agency should coordinate and support many essential clinical, developmental, and longitudinal research projects in transracial and transcultural adoption. There is an urgent need to serve these minority children in the best interests of their normal development and to help their adoptive families who are under stress.

REFERENCES

Baran, A., Sorosky, A., & Pannor, R. (1975). The dilemma of our adoptees. *Psychology Today, 9,* 98–100.

Berlin, I. N. (1978). Anglo-adoptions of native Americans: Repercussions in adolescence. *Child Psychiatry, 17,* 387–388.

Boys and Girls Aid Society. (1976). *National survey of black children adopted in 1974.* Portland, OR: Opportunity.

Care of Children Committee of Great Britain. (1946). Curtis Report. London: Her Majesty's Stationery Office.

Chestang, L. (1972). The dilemma of biracial adoption. *Social Work, 17,* 100–105.

Child Welfare League of America. (1968). *Standards for adoption service* (rev.). New York: Author.

Chimezie, A. (1975). Transracial adoption of black children. *Social Work, 20,* 296–301.

Clothier, F. (1939). Some aspects of problem adoption. *Orthopsychiatry, 9,* 598–615.

Cole, E. (1976). *Adoption Problems and Strategies 1976–1985.* Washington, DC: Children's Bureau, Office of Child Development. Department of Health, Education and Welfare.

Falk, L. L. (1969). Identity and the transracially adopted child. *Lutheran Social Welfare, Summer,* 18–25.

Falk, L. L. (1970). A comparative study of transracial and inracial adoptions. *Child Welfare, 49*(2), 82–88.

Fanshel, D. (1972). *Far from the reservation*. Metuchen, NJ: Scarecrow Press.

Feiertag, R. B. (1973). Committee on adoption and dependent care of American Academy of Pediatrics: Transracial adoption. *Pediatrics, 51*, 145–148.

Ferguson, M. (1969). *Inter-racial adoption: A comparative study*. Minneapolis, Minnesota.: University of Minnesota School of Social Work.

Fricke, H. (1965). Interracial adoption: The little revolution. *Social Work, 10*, 92–97.

Frisk, M. (1964). Identity problems and confused conceptions of the genetic ego in adopted children during adolescence. *Acta Paedopsychiatrica, 21*, 6–11.

Gallay, G. (1963). Interracial adoptions. *Canadian Welfare, 34*, 248–250.

Goodman, J. D., Silberstein, R. M., & Mandell, W. (1963). Adopted children brought to a child psychiatric clinic. *Archives of General Psychiatry, 9*, 451–456.

Goodman, M. E. (1964). *Race awareness in young children*. New York: Macmillan.

Grow, L. J., & Shapiro, D. (1974). *Black children, white parents: A study of transracial adoption*. New York: Child Welfare League of America.

Herzog, E. (1971). Some opinions of finding families for black children. *Children, 18*, 143–148.

Huard, L. A. (1956). The law of adoption: Ancient and modern. *Vanderbilt Law Review, 9*, 743–763.

Joe, B. (1978). In defense of intercountry adoption. *Social Service Review, 52*, 1–20.

Johnson, C. L. (1976). Transracial adoption: Victim of ideology. *Social Work, 21*, 241–243.

Jones, E. D. (1972). On transracial adoption of black children. *Child Welfare, 51*, 156–164.

Kim, S. P. (1980). Behavior symptoms in three transracially adopted Asian children: Diagnosis dilemma. *Child Welfare, 59*, 213–224.

Kim, S. P., Hong, S. D., & Kim, B. S. (1979). Adoption of Korean children by New York area couples: A preliminary study. *Child Welfare, 58*, 419–427.

Kirk, D. (1964). *Shared fate: A theory of adoption and mental health*. New York: Free Press of Glencoe.

Ladner, J. A. (1978). *Mixed families: Adopting across racial lines*. Garden City, NY: Anchor Books.

Lebo, J., Rogers, D., & Stuhlmann, C. (1965). *Adoptive placement of the Negro-Caucasian child*. Unpublished master's thesis, University of Minnesota, Minneapolis.

Madison, B. Q., & Schapiro, M. (1973). Black adoption—Issues and policies: Review of literature. *Social Service Review, 47*(4), 531–560.

McWhinnie, A. M. (1969). The adopted child in adolescence. In G. Caplan & S. Levovici (Eds.), *Psychological perspectives*. New York: Basic Books.

Mitchell, M. M. (1969). Transracial adoptions: Philosophy and practice. *Child Welfare, 48*, 613–619.

Moreland, J. K. (1969). Race awareness among American and Hong Kong Chinese children. *American Journal of Sociology, 75*, 360–374.

Peller, L. (1963). Further comment on adoption. *Bulletin of the Philadelphia Psychoanalytic Association, 13*, 1–14.

Presser, S. B. (1971). The historical background of the American law of adoption. *Journal of Family Law, 11*, 443–516.

Rathbun, C., DiVirgilio, L., & Waldfogel, S. (1958). The restitutive process in children following radical separation from family and culture. *American Journal of Orthopsychiatry, 28*, 408–415.

Rathbun, C., McLaughlin, H., Bennett, C., & Garland, J. A. (1965). Later adjustment of children following radical separation from family and culture. *American Journal of Orthopsychiatry, 35*, 604–609.

Schechter, M. D., Carlson, P. V., Simmons, J. Q., & Work, H. H. (1964). Emotional problems in the adoptee. *Archives of General Psychiatry, 10*, 109–118.

Sharrar, M. L. (1971). Attitude of black natural parents regarding adoption. *Child Welfare, 50*, 186–289.

Shibutani, J., & Kwan, K. (1965). *Ethnic stratification: A comparative approach.* New York: Macmillan.

Simon, R. J. (1974). An assessment of racial awareness, preference, and self-identity among white and adopted nonwhite children. *Social Problems, 22,* 43–57.

United States Department of Health, Education and Welfare. (1976). *Adoptions in 1976.* Washington, DC: National Center for Social Statistics.

United States Immigration and Naturalization Service. (1968–1975). *Annual reports.* Washington, DC: U.S. Government Printing Office.

Vieni, M. (1975). Transracial adoption is a solution now. *Social Work, 20,* 419–421.

Weider, H. (1977). On being told of adoption. *Psychoanalytic Quarterly, 46,* 1–12.

PART III

Parenting

Chapter 6

Working Mothers

Ruth L. Fuller

My interest in the concerns of the millions of working mothers in the United States has a long history. I am a working mother and come from a family of working mothers. During the past 25 years, in New York City and Denver, Colorado, the pleasures and conflicts of several hundred working mothers have been presented to me. These mothers represent a wide spectrum of ethnic, cultural, and educational backgrounds.

Whether patient, colleague, or friend, each is a participant in one of the most jarring influences on the American family in the decade: the marked shift in employment patterns of parents. The conventional ideal of the father working outside of the home while the mother remains a full-time homemaker has now become the exception rather than the rule. According to the United States Bureau of Census, by 1979, 14% of America's 59 million families lived in a traditional arrangement, while another 14.1% were headed by 2.3 million single mothers.

By 1980, 55.5% of all women who had children under 17 were employed. McFeatters (1981) has found that since World War II, the number of working women has increased 300% (more than 1 million per year) but that the number of working mothers has increased 1000%. From 1970 to 1979, *Working Mother* (Bulletin Board, 1980b) has reported, the faction of the American labor force with the greatest rate of increase has been married women with children under 6 years of age. By 1984, 45% of women with children under 1 year of age and 44% of women with children under 3 were employed outside the home, according to Young and Zigler (1986). Brazelton (1986) states that by 1990, it is expected that 70% of children will have two parents working outside the home. The patterns, influenced by choice but apparently forced by eco-

Ruth L. Fuller • Department of Psychiatry, University of Colorado Health Sciences Center, Denver, Colorado 80262.

nomic pressures, call for an adjustment in a common childrearing belief supported by such authors as Bowlby (1973) and Fraiberg (1977): that the best mothering—if not the only *good* mothering—is given by the mother herself.

Rooted in historical precedent, this belief has become entrenched in the American middle-class system, according to Hoffman and Nye (1974) and Nadelson and Notman (1981). The picture of two working parents has been associated with the working class or the working poor. It was assumed that the mother did not work unless the family could not survive otherwise. Often minority and immigrant extended families could become upwardly mobile only if two or more adults worked full time. The working-class goal was to achieve financial security so that the woman, whether or not she had children, did not have to work. Churchman (1981) reported a historical view of this process in a 1981 art exhibit on the roles of women in industrial America at the Smithsonian Museum of American History.

Individuals and groups of mothers have shared their views with me on hundreds of occasions. For example, a colleague, Rosalind, 37, frowned as she spoke of her history:

> I find it hard to believe that until I was twelve or thirteen years old, I did not know that my mother had been a high school teacher before she had children. She just stopped teaching at the beginning of her first pregnancy. When my seventh-grade English teacher stopped teaching because she was pregnant, I decided that I didn't want to be a teacher because I would either have to give up my career or have children but not both. Of course, I learned that teaching wasn't the cause of my dilemma but that bit of awareness came to me years after my "trauma."

Now the higher cost of living permits fewer families to maintain a middle-class standard on one salary; today the second income may only enable a family to simply break even rather than to get ahead (Aldous, 1982). The majority of mothers in the United States now work (Gottfried, 1988); thus, the assumption that the ideal mother is a full-time homemaker is being scrutinized with more care, as suggested by Hoffman and Nye (1974), Murray (1975), and Spurlock and Rembold (1978). Olds (1975) expresses the stronger view that exclusive mothering is probably unrealistic.

As the dependence on a second income grows, so does the value women and men place on the work itself. Until recent years, middle-class women often considered employment as a minor diversion from their major careers as homemakers. Kuzma's (1981) description of the ideal mother who did not work for money supports my finding from interviews with approximately 100 women who stated that temporary or part-time work might have added to the family income for luxuries, but

lucrative, full-time employment was unacceptable be.
were grown and out of the home.

Margaret, age 42, spoke to this point with humor:
worked part time, now and then, just for the extra goodies
family wanted. Of course, she did volunteer work all of the tim.
was very active in PTA projects, the Red Cross, Girl Scouts, any a.
that needed a volunteer. Now that I think about it, she must have
volunteered at least forty hours a week."

Today, lucrative part-time or temporary work may be scarce. Business and industry seek full-time employees who, once they have gained entry, will find it possible to advance within the company to greater responsibility, higher pay, and, presumably, greater personal satisfaction. Although job sharing is gaining in popularity, it remains the exception rather than the rule (Moskowitz & Townsend, 1989).

Through all career changes, the working mother remains responsible for her children. Some practical questions arise: How will my working hours be arranged? Who will care for my child? Other questions relate to profound issues of child development: How secure will my child feel? How well will my child learn? How will my children imagine themselves as adults and parents? Olds (1975) and Kuzma (1981) discuss other questions concerning the husband's feelings and the working mother's own goals. The questions—practical and profound—stem from one concern, the adequacy of mothering by a woman who works (Gottfried, 1988).

A common complaint from professional parents is lack of time; they must constantly set and revise priorities and examine the amount and quality of time that they devote to childrearing. Most women in the current force of working mothers were raised by mothers who were full-time homemakers, as noted by Belasco (unpublished paper) and Hoffman and Nye (1974). Working mothers' concern about the number of hours required for child care was the subject of an early study by Fisher in 1939. As summarized by Hoffman and Nye, the study showed that on an hourly basis, professional mothers spent as much actual time with their school-age children as did the full-time homemaker.

It is my impression that the time the nonworking mother spends at home while the children are in school, playing out-of-doors, or visiting a friend is inaccurately counted as active child care. It would be more accurate to regard this time as being "on call" (Fuller, unpublished paper, 1980). The working parent is also "on call," but from a job site instead of from home.

Formerly, it was expected that the full-time homemaker would have various social and volunteer commitments that required her to leave home, yet apparently American society weighed her availability to re-

..n home differently from that of the paid working parent. The difference between the opportunity for direct parent–child interaction and actual quality time spent is most important. Quality time devoted to child care has allowed working parents to more easily accommodate their job and childrearing responsibilities. Olds and Kuzma stress this point. Hoffman and Nye have summarized two studies that demonstrate that working mothers (1) plan more activities with their children than do nonworking mothers and (2) are more likely to seize the opportunity for additional, spontaneous activities.

A colleague, Maria, 38, was responding to her 3-year-old daughter, Karen's, request to look at family pictures with her. Maria had numerous business calls to make but "seized the moment" to spend some quality time with Karen. As mother and daughter turned to Maria's rather stern passport photograph, Karen looked puzzled and asked, "Why isn't Mommy smiling?" Maria harbored a secret concern that returning to work in an administrative position might be depriving and damaging her daughter. Maria believed that she was a good mother most of the time, but she had her doubts. She was rightfully delighted to see her daughter's joyous perception of her mother: a happy, smiling face and a woman content with her life, her child, and her work.

Another example was presented by a friend who is an accomplished businesswoman. Laura, 35, was working on a budget for her company. The work needed to be finished within 48 hours and she felt pressed. Her 2 ½-year-old daughter, Anne, was sitting at her feet playing with her toys. Anne looked up at her mother and asked for the legal pad on the desk. After getting the pad, Anne took a pencil and made a series of scribbles and giggled. "What are you making?" the concerned mother asked. Anne beamed, saying, "Budget, budget, budget." Laura felt relieved and then shared in Anne's pleasure. As a businesswoman and mother, she gave herself a well-deserved vote of confidence. She was spending quality time with her daughter and meeting her professional deadline.

The working mothers that I have treated as a psychiatrist are in pain. Most often they came to consult with me as a child psychiatrist. They usually describe their children as unhappy or not doing well in school. The mothers have been accurate in describing the children but inaccurate in attributing the cause to maternal employment per se (Gottfried & Gottfried, 1988). Frequently, the children were unhappy because the mothers were depressed and distant, not because their mothers worked. Over recent years, more single working mothers have contacted me with concerns about themselves. Common complaints are of fatigue, confusion, lethargy, sadness, insomnia, guilt about working, and doubt about their abilities as mothers. The most frequent diagnosis is of depression. I have observed a range of personality disorders; of these, dependent, avoidant, and compulsive disorders are the most common.

Whether presenting an initial concern about a child or about themselves, both married and single mothers have expressed feelings of guilt about working, although nearly all of them work out of necessity. Individual, couple, and/or family therapy would be offered to the working mother. Many working mothers initially choose individual interviews for themselves and then opt for family therapy. This preference for family therapy supports the Poznanski, Maxey, and Marsden (1974) view that the mutual interplay of intrapsychic and external factors is important. The family members renegotiate the problems of who needs care from whom and under what circumstances. The working mother reexamines her guilt and clarifies issues for herself. Since most working mothers work out of necessity, their guilt is associated with the assumption that mothers should provide a different (better, more affluent) environment for their children. In Anderson's discussion (1983) of the Bodin and Mitelman book on working mothers, the theme of guilt is present even though 88% of the mothers did not wish to be full-time homemakers. If the mother is working by choice and feels guilty, she needs to reexamine her feelings about the choice. Professional working mothers have been encouraged in their convictions by a number of supports. They receive recognition in their fields, can decide what steps to make in a career ladder, and make more money as professionals. More middle-class mothers are working out of necessity. Working-class mothers usually have never known a time of not working. Their feelings are illustrated by this vignette.

> A group of working black mothers who were both married and single came for a group session. Inez, a divorced mother of three young children, asked Sonia, a widowed mother of five young adult sons and daughters, how she had managed to raise her children with so little money. Inez said, "My mother worked all my life and is still working. My grandmother just stopped working at seventy. I feel so tired now. I might as well give up now rather than wait fifty years." Sonia leaned over and took the younger woman's hand. "Inez, you need some help! You're talking as though you have to do everything yourself. You've got family. You've got friends. Don't be ashamed to say that you need help. After my husband died, I had help from my family and friends who were just like family. Kids know that if you could make the world different for them you would—you love them—but you ain't no Superhero! The kids put in their share too because they know you love them and they love you. You didn't ask, 'God, please make me broke all the time!' You're teaching your children what I taught mine: good common sense, faith in themselves and each other, nobody owes you a living, things that they need to make it in this world. Each of us, we do the best we can. Nobody does better than their best and nobody's best is the same as anybody else's."

Although I do not have a formal follow-up treatment survey, I have a significant follow-up through the networking of referrals made by working mothers. These mothers found therapy helpful in resolving conflicts and regaining confidence. After therapy they were able to more thoroughly enjoy their children and their jobs.

In addition to concerns about her children, a married working mother is concerned about her marriage. In 1982 Morall and Fuller presented this question to a group of 35 professional women at the Colorado Annual Women in Business Conference. All of the women agreed that setting and revising priorities were crucial to maintaining good parenting and a successful career. A surprising finding was the unanimous statement by married mothers that they saw their husbands as equally important as a parent and that the amount of parenting shared with their husbands was a crucial factor in their feeling confident that their children received good parenting.

A larger view of the feelings that husbands have is seen in Anderson's (1983) summary of the Bodin and Mitelman work. Of 442 working mothers, only 20% believed that their husbands would prefer a full-time homemaker. More than 33% reported that they receive support from their husbands; a majority felt that their husbands were proud of them.

Nevertheless, women appear to maintain the central position of the manager in the home. In my practice, I found that couples who came into therapy had not been able to negotiate the changes in the running of the household that the mother's employment demanded. Hinebaugh's (1982) study on male attitudes toward equal childrearing found that men gave a 47% commitment effort overall. However, this effort was generally devoted to traditional male-role activity. One couple in treatment gave the following story which supports this finding:

> Gene, 32, and Cara, 30, had been working out a plan for sharing child care and housekeeping responsibilities. Cara was trying to be supportive of Gene but added an important complaint when she said, "Gene does spend time with the kids as soon as he gets home and before he leaves for work. He takes them out and plays with them. I put them to bed and get them up, dressed and to the sitter. That part [of the sharing] works fine. It is the housekeeping that doesn't work. He doesn't do laundry, dishes, dust, cook or clean. I have it all and I work just as many hours as he does." Gene agreed that Cara's picture was accurate.

The husbands in therapy often felt neglected and/or betrayed by their wives. They had assumed that mothers would always be full-time caregivers. They often had difficulty with the prospect of staying home with a sick child or seeing the mother's job as having a higher priority. Couples who work as partners have presented less competitiveness and appear less conflicted about sharing or delegating responsibilities for child care, housekeeping, and work. Cath, Gurwitt, and Ross (1982) have discussed the roles of fathers; the responses of husbands have been discussed by Olds (1975).

Let's look at the response shown by one husband in treatment. Sam, 39, became angry as he spoke. "If my wife didn't work, we wouldn't be able to make ends meet. We both know that. She works hard all day and then is terrific with the kids. I don't know how she does it. I'm really proud of her, but I don't know how I would take it if she made more money than me. I still feel that the man is supposed to provide for his family. No sir, I don't know how I would take it."

A reasonable guess would be that Sam would not "take it" too well unless he could change his assumption that a man's worth is measured by the number of dollars in his paycheck. Men who share Sam's feelings may not be as vocal as the growing number of men who want to be more involved with child care and homemaking. The Boston Women's Health Book Collective (1978) contains vignettes about fathers who wish for more time with their children.

Nadelson and Notman's (1981) survey of the literature and discussion of the difference between maternal absence and maternal deprivation reaches an important conclusion. They summarize studies that point to the infant's ability to make multiple attachments to father and other caregivers. The authors add that separation from the mother is not the same as distancing between mother and child. Cox (1975) has looked at the effects of the combination of father absence and working mothers on children and found father absence to be significant. Warshaw (1976) has studied the impact of working mothers on children and found no measurable effect. Rosenthal (1978) has studied working and nonworking mothers in intact and nonintact homes. Children in intact and nonintact homes have the same perception of mothers, Rosenthal reports, but children of divorce perceive fathers as least demanding. Children whose parents are separated perceive fathers as most rejecting.

Other selected child development studies deal with how children view their mothers' working. Brookins (1978) has studied a sample of black middle- and working-class children to assess how maternal employment affected their concepts of sex roles and occupational choices. After searching the literature, Brookins found only two other studies that involved black children; all other studies involved white children. The literature search revealed that children of working mothers generally show more approval of maternal employment, more flexibility in their concepts of sex roles, and a higher evaluation of women's competence than do children of nonworking mothers. She did note (with caution because of the small sample of 36 families) that social class did not turn out to be a predictable variable in determining the children's view of their working mothers.

> In a support group, 14 professional women were discussing their children's perception of mother. Anne, 38, a lawyer, spoke of her daughter, Sharon, age 10, and her comments to a playmate. "My mom has to read a lot of books and write a lot of papers. She goes to court to explain to the judge what she needs to do and why. So, we can't play at my house tomorrow because court is in session. If the case is finished by Friday, you can spend the weekend. My Mom is quite important to a lot of people too."

Sharon's comment points to a positive result of maternal employment, the child's experience of acquiring greater independence in making choices about activities at an earlier age. Olds (1975) notes that the working mother is more likely to feel pressured by tight schedules than is the full-time homemaker; thus, the working mother may welcome her child's moves toward independence. Households have their individual systems for encouraging independence appropriate to the various stages of childhood. Full-time working mothers may encourage their children's self-reliance earlier than do nonworking mothers. Working mothers may stress the importance of activities such as going to school with peers or alone and may trust their children to carry a front-door key, use the stove, and make judgments about handling their time. The full-time homemaker may derive less pleasure from witnessing her children make these independent steps toward maturity and may feel that her children do not need her anymore. Brookins (1978), Hoffman and Nye (1974), and Nadelson and Notman (1981) note this finding in their searches of the literature.

> During a women's group, Thelma, 30, mother of three, shared her struggles with the issue of her children's independence. "My children are very close in age—Donna, 10, Rick, 9, and Mike, 8. I really struggle with the question of having them go to a sitter every day after school. The kids came to me and told me that they were bigger. Donna knows how to cook well. Rick and Mike know their chores too. They remind me that they like their home and they behave 'real good.' They know all of the rules of safety in answering the door. They use the sitter, across the hall, to 'check on' them. I began to think about how pleased they were when they left for school on their own and Donna got her door key because she was responsible. They had dinner fixed when I got home so that I could see how well they could do. They convinced me that it was time to let go of them a little more and I felt proud of them. Now Mike is the first one to say 'we need more mothering' or 'that's enough motherness.' "

This view is different from the historical perspective, reported by Raybon (1983), that regarded the "latchkey" children as totally deprived. "Street kids" who take care of themselves have been seen as totally neglected. Spurlock and Rembold (1978) have anticipated this controversy. The collective child care that occurs informally in the neighborhood (or "in the street" in dense urban areas such as New York City's Harlem) when the oldest child or adolescent takes charge and the handiest neighborhood parent helps to supervise can still prove to be positive, resourceful, and adaptive child care (Fuller, unpublished paper, 1981).

Between 1966 and 1978, I became familiar with the informal patterns of child care in East Harlem and Central Harlem. A 9-year-old girl explained the street-based child care system to me. Rhoda said:

> My dad's at work at the garage. His number is 234-1511. My mom's at work at the phone company. Her number is 858-1177. My sister gets home from high school before I get home. I get something to eat; she goes to work at the restaurant around the corner at four o'clock. Her number is 973-6670. My big brother is supposed to be home at four o'clock, but he usually goes to see his girlfriend, but she lives in the next [apartment], building number four C. I play with Aisha almost every day because she's nice. I don't play with bad kids but nobody messes with me either. If I need anything, I ask Aisha's mother first. She's a nice mother but she likes to feed me too many vegetables! Sometimes, when my mother is at home on vacation she looks out for Aisha too. My sister is always at the restaurant, so if I need to, I go there and wait for her to get finished. Now, if I am sick, either my mother or my sister, sometimes my brother, once even my father, stays with me. You got that? Do you want me to explain it again?

Rhoda felt well cared for in this complex but clearly defined system. Her mother said she felt that her child was safe, without a center for latchkey children as was started in Acton, Massachusetts (Escape, 1983). A working mother who has confidence that her child is well cared for in her absence will probably have fewer doubts about her performance as a mother. A majority of working mothers opt for care somewhat more structured than the informal street arrangement previously described, yet a mother searching for day care may find that no consistent and generally available method exists (Young & Zigler, 1986). Simons and Strauss (1981) noted in 1981 that 1.1 million openings existed for the 7 million children under 6 years of age. Phillips (1983) describes the waiting period for child care as being 18 to 24 months in 1985. At the same time, the most rapid increase in maternal employment was seen in mothers with children under the age of 2 years.

The number of options for child care vary with the work hours, geographic location of the family, proximity of relatives, other support systems, parent income, and absolute minimum requirements that the parent deems necessary for the child's care. If we consider the work hours first, we must try to determine how much child care is necessary. As the labor market demands more full-time employment, we can assume that 7- to 10-hour days of child care will become more common. If the child is in school, is there a need for supervision before and after school? Another decision to be made is whether child care will be given in or outside the home.

At one time or another, I have used nearly all of the arrangements described. For most parents, employment of a full-time professional housekeeper is not a real option. Such professionals are extremely expensive. Although novice housekeepers command a lesser salary, parents are often understandably reluctant to grant major or total responsibility to such inexperienced or untrained individuals.

A live-in housekeeper is also a financial impossibility for most parents. It may be true that there are still career live-in housekeepers, but often this occupation is temporary employment for a person who is training for another profession. For example, I met Elise, a young woman that I had known as a college student. She was escorting two children to a nearby park. She went on to explain. "I had planned to go to graduate school right after college but I didn't have the money. I took this job so that I would have a place to live while I made and saved money. I estimate that I will need to work six to eight months in order to save enough, and then I will leave."

Elise's employers were pleased with this bright, resourceful, and friendly young woman, but soon they would have to begin the search for a new housekeeper. A variation on the live-in arrangement that has worked well for some parents is *au pair* living with a student. The *au pair* arrangement works well if the young man or woman is mature and has flexible hours that the parents need.

The Dillon family described their very happy experience living near a university. Bernice, the mother, began: "We found that we needed to work out an arrangement with students who were in the liberal arts rather than the sciences. I could adjust my work days because I needed child care after school and again in the evening for a class. The science majors tended to be busy at three or four p.m. Leslie [the student] enjoyed being with the children. She had been sitting with children since she was twelve years old. We had a very tearful good-bye when she graduated."

Andy, age 7, added: "Leslie was fun but you had to do your work too. I hope that the next sitter will be fun too and like to play ball."

Other couples have been disappointed with this system. Marsha, a physician, spoke for her family. "We felt as though we had taken on the supervision of still another child, an adolescent, rather than obtaining the child care that we needed. Meg [the student] would have trouble with her classwork, boyfriend, or her mother, and I would spend hours trying to help her decide what she was going to do about the problem. It was exhausting. One day she was 'overwhelmed' and did not meet my child at the nursery. Worse still, she didn't call to tell me. I knew that the 'arrangement' had just ended."

Siegel-Gorelick (1983) found that approximately 40% of parents use part-time day care for their children in their own home. The concern of the working parent in this situation is: "What do I do if the caregiver doesn't come?" The parent's ability to work in a predictable manner depends on the caregiver's own ability to work. Vacations, illness, weather, and travel conditions are factors that influence the caregiver's availability, which, in turn, influences the working parent.

There was a phone call recently from a colleague, Alicia. "Quick, tell me if you know any sitters! My regular caregiver just called in sick and my backup person is on vacation. My neighbor isn't at home and I need to be in the office in two hours!"

Sometimes the most carefully laid plans fall apart. The dearth and high cost of housekeepers or in-home caregivers make family day care the choice of approximately 45% of working mothers. Family day care services may or may not be licensed by a state agency such as the Social Services Department. Women who provide day care are usually mothers themselves. Young women who provide day care often have children of their own who are part of the group of three to five children that are cared for daily. Older day care mothers usually have children who are in school or are adults.

The day care mother offers a planned day. The cost is generally higher in the northeast and west coast regions. Usually, there is a room or an area of the home reserved for the children. Most day care mothers have child-sized furniture, but they may ask the working mother to bring any special equipment. Generally, it is found that the smaller the number of children in a day care home, the more flexible the schedule for the day. When there are eight or more children, a more structured schedule tends to be followed.

The usual day starts with the arrival of the children, indoor play with toys, perhaps a group activity such as drawing or viewing selected educational TV programs. After a snack, the children play in the yard or in a nearby park, eat lunch, take a nap, and then have another period of indoor or outdoor play or a trip (for a smaller group). This activity is followed by snack and free play until the children leave. As Galinsky and Hooks (1979) and Siegel-Gorelick (1983) have written, day care parents rightfully see themselves as professionals and work hard at improving their skills. I have found that family day care fathers are few in number and are usually part of a day care couple. Siegel-Gorelick has reported similar findings.

The members of extended families frequently share child care: Some parents work while another parent or grandparent takes full responsibility for the children collectively. As with the other informal day care arrangements, relatives do not tend to see themselves as engaged in a difficult profession. Furthermore, I (Fuller, 1985) have found that such family arrangements have been undervalued in their adaptive function and have even been considered pathological in the dominant culture of American society. Working parents who ask members of the original extended family for child care have been accused of being unable to separate from their own parents or parental figures.

Another mental health professional, Angela, 40, called me. She sounded distressed and explained why. "I was talking with friends at work this morning and mentioned that I was very pleased that my mother was coming to live with us and would be taking care of the children. I was delighted that the children would get to know their grandmother and that my mother would have the pleasure of taking care of them. She is a wonderful mother. She loves children. I was stunned, hurt, then confused when everyone in the room attacked me as 'immature' and 'still struggling with separation issues' because my mother is coming! David [her husband] and I had thought about this plan for a long time. We weighed the change in living style for my mother, the reorganization of our household, the change in privacy, and even the financial gain for everyone. It never occurred to me that my colleagues and friends would be so, so prejudiced!"

I (Fuller, 1985) have suggested that with the change in life-styles, employment patterns, and living situations, the reestablishment of extended families should become more widespread. These extended families may be new ones or old ones, and may occupy one shared living unit or several in close proximity.

Group day care or nursery schools provide options for some working parents, but cost, space limitations, and scheduling may preclude these resources from helping others (Belasco, unpublished paper, 1978). Many parents find themselves ineligible for group day care sponsored by public funds because a two-income family makes too much money (Triggs, personal communication, 1978). In 1983 the cost for each child is $5–6/day and $10–11/day for each infant or toddler (Siegel-Gorelick, 1983). Gamble and Zigler (1986) project a much higher cost of up to $150/week for quality infant day care.

Approximately 18% of children receiving day care are in day care centers, according to Siegel-Gorelick. The centers have larger numbers of children than the typical family child-care home. Siegel-Gorelick describes the day care center as technically having no curriculum and thus differing from the nursery school; however, that technicality is misleading. As a consultant to a dozen day care centers in New York and Denver, I have been impressed with the teachers' curriculum plans, educational goals, and evaluation methods. They take pleasure in seeing youngsters in their programs develop their full preschool talents in anticipation of starting the first grade. I do agree that there is a range in planning and quality of care in centers across the country. In 1983 the United States Bureau of Census listed 656 day care centers in Colorado alone. The need for greater uniformity in the quality of day care is addressed by Phillips (1983) in her discussion of the 1985 Federal Model Child Care Standards Act. Individual variables might be assessed as McCartney (1982) did in studying language development in day care children in nine centers. Working parents who participate in or establish a cooperative child care center or a baby-sitting exchange (Douglas & Jason, 1986) find that the cost is less because each family contributes time toward the care of the children.

Working Mother (Bulletin Board, 1980c) has described an innovative program in Orlando, Florida, called 4-C (Community Coordinated Child Care for Central Florida). Parents who use 4-C are charged a sliding fee. They receive a voucher that can be used for the child care option of the parents' choice. Providers are paid by 4-C from its pooled financial resources. From 1971 to 1980, 4-C served 3,000 children.

A less formal cooperative arrangement is accomplished when several friends rotate care of their collective children. Still other working mothers are usually referred to as baby-sitters rather than family day caregivers because it is less likely that the neighbors or friends see themselves as child care professionals. Other community organizations, such as Montview Boulevard Presbyterian Church in Denver, provide child care for members of the surrounding community in a program called Parents' Morning Out (Taylor, personal communication, 1985). Whether using the licensed, unlicensed, co-op, or informal day care setting, the working mother needs to feel that the child's care will be consistent and harmonious with parental care.

For the self-employed, family-employed, or autonomous executive professional woman, child care may be given at the business office. For example, after a candid staff meeting of the mental health clinic I co-directed, we set a policy that allowed all staff working mothers to bring children to work with them. I preferred having mother and child at work rather than absenteeism. The working mothers used this option selectively for surprisingly brief periods of time. The option was most appreciated by mothers of infants who were not yet walking. The mothers' decided preference for toddlers was in-home or family day care. For nursery school and school-age children, school near home was the only preference. Before this experiment at the worksite, each staff person had assumed that there would be enough employee need to justify job-site child care. We concluded that a reasonable choice of options was most desirable. Olds (1975) and Siegel-Gorelick (1983) reported similar findings.

The possibility of using the office for child care decreases markedly in the general business world. Siegel-Gorelick (1983) reported that some businesses, such as Stride Rite (Massachusetts), have established child care for their employees. Employee demand for this option is resulting in increasing availability of jobsite child care (Moskowitz & Townsend, 1989). The model is usually not cooperative since the mothers, and occasionally the fathers, would not be able to take turns on a truly cooperative basis. Employers may simply allow parents to occasionally bring an infant or child to their place of business for the day.

The most common complaint voiced by working parents is the lack of affordable, predictable, quality day care. Unfortunately, children are often shuttled to two or more settings over the course of the week. As Mark, age 5, said to me, "I wish that every day was Wednesday because that's the day that Jeannie keeps me. I don't like Friday because that's the day that Roberta keeps me. The other days Nana [his grandmother] keeps me."

If a parent has a shift in schedule, the arrangements are even more complex. When a child becomes ill, care outside of the home may not be feasible. If the child is seriously ill, parents must decide which one of them will stay at home. The ingenuity and resourcefulness of the working mother in making these complex arrangements cannot be overemphasized. One concern that parents and mental health professionals have shared is that the very complexity of the arrangements often leads to several child care figures who appear sequentially and/or concurrently during the child's life, and that such an experience may be detrimental to the child's development.

With relatively recent research into the role of the father and other important caregivers as reviewed by Nadelson and Notman (1981), the past assumption that the existence of several caregivers is bad for children is being reexamined. Today fathers have begun to figure more prominently in the child care scheme and child development (Cath et al., 1982), including the role of single parent, as noted by Anderson (1983), the Boston Women's Health Book Collective (1978), Hinebaugh (1982), Lowenstein (1977), and Simons and Strauss (1981). When both married parents work, the father may have to change his perception of what a family should be. There is greater demand for sharing in the care of the home and in child care, with the exception of a minority of couples who can afford to have a full-time professional assume these responsibilities. Greater sharing deepens the relationship between father and child. The child has two parents who are intimately familiar with his or her day-to-day care; stress develops when these new roles are not clearly defined. I have already referred to a potential difficulty that may arise when parents must decide who will stay home with an ill child. Much depends on whose care the child would prefer, as well as flexibility of work hours and demand of each parent's job. Investigators must continue gathering more data about these relationships as employment patterns and family life continue to change (Gottfried & Gottfried, 1988).

We have looked at some of the issues related to the impact of work patterns on the American family. The working couple now dominates the country's labor force. Child care problems, which formerly afflicted only working class and working poor, have now become the concern of the average American family.

What are the prospects for the future? From an economic point of view, supporting a family on one parent's income in a two-parent home will become more and more a luxury. The two-parent working family will probably remain the norm (Brazelton, 1986). In 1980 the median income of a single working mother was less than half of the median income for an American family. At that time Cadden (1980) rightfully asked how single mothers manage. If these patterns continue, the extended family may be reconstituted under one roof again in larger segments of society.

For example, while I was working with one group of 40 graduate students, 6 described their move back to the parental home in order to attend graduate school. All 6 earned some income, but all agreed that they could not afford to maintain a separate residence and attend school simultaneously. One student shared the information that a disturbing number of his friends were now returning home (or not leaving) because they did not have jobs.

In many ethnic groups, the extended family has been maintained throughout the history of American society. It may be that child care would naturally unfold in such settings involving group living, but for the family that maintains a separate dwelling and makes its own care arrangements, there is a persistent need for flexibility in work hours, for accessible, quality day care at affordable prices, for more discretionary use of sick and annual leave to allow for child care, and for postpartum coverage for the minimal time that working mothers are on leave. The most common postpartum coverage figures that I have heard reported by patients and colleagues extends from several weeks to 6 months.

These supports for working mothers already exist in other countries, such as Sweden. In 1980 *Working Mother* (Bulletin Board, 1980a) summarized a then-new Swedish law. Both mothers and fathers may obtain up to 18 months of leave. The employee is given 90% of her or his salary for 9 months and then is on leave without pay for up to 9 more months. Either parent may then decrease the hours in the workday to 6 until the child finishes the first year of school or is 8 years old.

The relative lack of supports in American society may be influenced by a number of factors. First, we have witnessed a lag time in public acceptance of the fact that working parents are the rule rather than the exception and in realization that current employment trends are not temporary. Second, the prospect of government-sponsored child care evokes fears of socialism and greater fragmentation of the family. In the current political climate of decentralization of resources and authority, working mothers are truly concerned that their inadequate resources may shrink further. Working mothers are concerned that their prospects in the labor force may continue to be as McFeatters reported in 1981: The typical working woman is 34 years old, needs to work, and will do so often at the bottom of the labor market for 27.6 years.

Psychiatrists have been encouraged to support mothers in their own identity. Working mothers ask for tangible supports in addition to therapeutic support. Head (1979) describes a unique, tangible support to single parents in Denver, Colorado. Warren Village is a 90-family apartment facility for single parents that has been in operation since 1974. In its first 5 years of operation, 461 families with 700 children were served. In approximately 1984, Warren Village II was opened.

Shrier, Buxtom, and Brodkin (1982) considered the problems of parenting and work difficult enough to merit a course for first-year medical students. Belasco (unpublished paper, 1978) added an argument that information be shared with working parents in general.

The American employment tradition has required that employees fit the demands of work rather than that employment settings accommodate family needs. With the advent of increasingly flexible work hours forced by energy conservation, commuter flow, and employee demand, some of the necessary changes may be evolving. Nevertheless, the needs of working mothers are pressing; child care and mental health professionals as well as employers must address the fact that the first generation of American children to be raised by a majority of working mothers is here. As Brazelton (1986) reminds us, it will take a generation to fully appreciate the impact that this change in child care has had on our citizens. Gottfried and Gottfried (1988) point to the method of assessing the impact of this change—namely, longitudinal studies in the context of family processes and employment variables and controlled for extraneous variables. In 1988 Gottfried and Gottfried found that across the studies they reviewed, "the overwhelming finding obtained was that maternal employment *per se* was not significantly related to children's development."

References

Aldous, J. (Ed.). (1982). *Two paychecks: Life in dual-earner families.* Beverly Hills, CA: Sage.
Anderson, J. (1983). Working mothers wouldn't turn back. *Rocky Mountain News,* July 11, p. 40.

Boston Women's Health Book Collective, The. (1978). *Ourselves and our children.* New York: Random House.

Bowlby, J. (1973). *Attachment and loss* (Vol. 2). New York: Basic Books.

Brazelton, T. B. (1986). Issues for working parents. *American Journal of Orthopsychiatry, 56,* 14–25.

Brookins, G. (1978). *Maternal employment: Its impact on the sex roles and occupational choices of middle working class black children.* Doctoral dissertation, Harvard University.

Bulletin Board. (1980a). The work world. *Working Mother, 3* (January), 8.

Bulletin Board. (1980b). The work world. *Working Mother, 3* (May), 30.

Bulletin Board. (1980c). The home front. *Working Mother, 3* (July), 8.

Cadden, V. (1980). How do single mothers manage on less than $10,000 a year? *Working Mother, 3* (May), 41.

Cath, S. H., Gurwitt, A. G., & Ross, J. M. (1982). *Father and child: Developmental and clinical perspectives.* Boston: Little, Brown.

Churchman, D. (1981). Exhibit traces working woman in United States. *Rocky Mountain News,* December 9, p. 2-M.

Cox, M. (1975). *The effects of father absence and working mothers on children.* Doctoral dissertation, University of Virginia.

Douglas, J. A., & Jason, L. A. (1986). Building social support systems through a babysitting exchange program. *American Journal of Orthopsychiatry, 56,* 103–108.

Escape from "latchkey syndrome." (1983). *Rocky Mountain News,* July 4, p. 49.

Fraiberg, S. (1977). *Every child's birthright.* New York: Basic Books.

Fuller, R. L. (1985). Adoption, foster care, day care, and other living arrangements. In R. C. Simons (Ed.), *Understanding human behavior in health and illness* (3rd ed.). Baltimore: Williams & Wilkins.

Galinsky, E., & Hooks, W. H. (1979). A home away from home. *Working Mother, 2,* 103.

Gamble, T. J., & Zigler, E. (1986). Effects of infant day care: Another look at the evidence. *American Journal of Orthopsychiatry, 56,* 26–42.

Gottfried, A. E. (1988). Maternal employment and children's development: An introduction of issues. In A. E. Gottfried & A. W. Gottfried (Eds.), *Maternal employment and children's development* (pp. 3–8). New York: Plenum Press.

Gottfried, A. E., & Gottfried, A. W. (1988). Maternal employment and children's development: An integration of longitudinal findings with implications for social policy. In A. E. Gottfried & A. W. Gottfried (Eds.), *Maternal employment and children's development* (pp. 269–289). New York: Plenum Press.

Head, T. (1979). Starting over. *Working Mother, 2* (November), 85.

Hinebaugh, F. (1982). *Male attitudes toward equality between the sexes and desired allocation of child-rearing tasks.* Doctoral dissertation, Michigan State University.

Hoffman, L. W., & Nye, F. I. (1974). *Working Mothers.* San Francisco: Jossey-Bass.

Kuzma, K. (1981). *Working Mothers* (2nd ed.). Los Angeles: Stratford Press.

Lowenstein, J. (1977). *A comparison of self-esteem between boys living with single-parent mothers and boys living with single-parent fathers.* Doctoral dissertation, University of Maryland.

McCartney, K. (1982). *The effect of quality of day care environment upon children's language development.* Doctoral dissertation, Yale University.

McFeatters, D. (1981). Work profile: Women face low-paid, dead-end jobs. *Rocky Mountain News,* January 20, p. 46.

Moskowitz, M., & Townsend, C. (1989). The 60 best companies in America for working mothers. *Working Mother, 12* (October), 74–100.

Murray, A. (1975). Maternal employment reconsidered. *American Journal of Orthopsychiatry, 45,* 773–790.

Nadelson, C., & Notman, M. (1981). Child psychiatry perspectives: Women, work, and children. *Journal of the American Academy of Child Psychiatry, 20,* 863–875.

Olds, S. W. (1975). *The mother who works outside the home.* New York: Child Study Press.

Phillips, D. (1983). The federal model child care standards act of 1985: Step in the right direction or hollow gesture. *American Journal of Orthopsychiatry, 56,* 56–64.

Poznanski, E., Maxey, A., & Marsden, G. (1974). Parental adaptations to maternal employment. *Journal of the American Academy of Child Psychiatry, 13,* 319–334.

Raybon, P. (1983). Feelings of fear linger for latchkey kids. *Rocky Mountain News,* July 4, p. 48.

Rosenthal, D. (1978). *Working and non-working mothers in intact and nonintact families and effects on the child's perception of the parent-child relationship, educational achievement, self-concept, occupational aspirations and vocational maturity.* Doctoral dissertation, State University of New York at Buffalo.

Shrier, D., Buxtom, M., & Brodkin, A. (1982). Parenting and professionalism: A course for first-year medical students. *Journal of the American Academy of Child Psychiatry, 21,* 575–578.

Siegel-Gorelick, B. (1983). *The working parent's guide to child care.* Boston: Little, Brown.

Simons, R. C., & Strauss, D. (1981). Marital dysfunction, separation and divorce. In R. C. Simons & H. Pardes (Eds.), *Understanding human behavior in health and illness* (2nd ed.). Baltimore: Williams & Wilkins.

Spurlock, J., & Rembold, K. (1978). Women at fault: Societal stereotypes and clinical conclusions. *Journal of the American Academy of Child Psychiatry, 17,* 383–386.

Warshaw, R. (1976). *The effects of working mothers on children.* Doctoral dissertation, Adelphi University.

Young, K. T., & Zigler, E. (1986). Infant and toddler day care: Regulations and policy implications. *American Journal of Orthopsychiatry, 56,* 43–55.

Chapter 7

Mothers of Exceptional Children

MARY S. AKERLEY

> *I came to the conclusion that it has definitely altered my parenting, and that*
> *when the autistic child is the first child—you are just learning parenting for*
> *the very first time, you are unsure of who you are as a parent—and you are*
> *learning the ropes with a defective educational toy.*
> CONNIE TORISKY, National Society for Autistic Children

Connie Torisky and I have sons with autism; hers is the oldest of four children, mine is the youngest. What follows is a reflection on that experience. Although autism is a relatively rare disability, I believe my reflection has validity for any mother of a disabled child.

IMAGES OF MOTHERHOOD

From the time a little girl receives her first baby doll, she begins to develop her internal image of herself as a mother. The doll itself has a lot to do with how the image is formed: It is pretty, it is healthy in appearance, and—at least while reasonably new—has both eyes and all four appendages. It cries and sometimes even speaks on cue. It eats, wets, walks exactly as Dr. Spock decrees it should.

Nothing in this marvelous training tool prepares a girl later to mother a defective child. Nothing in the development of her internal self-image has allowed for mothering a child who is mute or blind, retarded or crippled, deaf or autistic. If the baby doll loses a leg, it is either fixed (usually by Daddy) or ignored. Mother-love-in-training simply remembers baby as it was in its gift box glory. If a handicapped child actually existed in our little girl's world, it was in all likelihood hidden away. The American dream does not include the imperfect.

MARY S. AKERLEY • Sasscer, Clagett, Channing & Bucher, Upper Marlboro, Maryland 20772.

DEALING WITH DISABILITIES

In short, the effect of the birth of a handicapped child on its mother can fairly be described as culture shock; this is true to some extent even if the newborn is perfectly normal. It cries and wets on its own cues, not its mother's, but even that shock is cushioned somewhat by previous experience. The new mother has, in all probability, done some baby-sitting in her teens and some reading during her pregnancy. She also has access to a pediatrician or a well-baby clinic, both sources of help and assurance, and—if her baby is normal—she has peer support. Most women have friends or neighbors with whom to compare notes or from whom to seek advice. That traditional support system is likely to break down, however, when a handicapped child is born. The mother can find a new system of external supports, but she must deal with an altered set of internal values first.

When our "ideal" parent is confronted with a real-life, diaper-soil-ing, howling baby, some adjustments are usually made quickly. Harder adjustments come later when the confrontation is with a teenager deal-ing with the complications of adolescent life. Adjustments, perforce, are made anew with each baby (and teenager). It is in making these adjust-ments that the parental self is created. From that perspective, parenting a handicapped child can be viewed as the extreme of the norm; it simply requires adjustment on a grander scale. A child rarely lives up to its parents' expectations; a handicapped child's areas of departure are just more obvious, much earlier in life. Unfortunately, the new mother is not allowed that simple reasoning because her child's difference is identified not as uniqueness but as deviance.

Part of what we call deviance is based on mass cultural values that are so ingrained in the society that they exist independently of any individual. However, the reverse is, of course, not true. The individual members of a society develop and evaluate themselves and others in terms of those values. It takes tremendous inner strength and self-confi-dence to reject those values consciously and live independently of them. Most of a "handicapped mother's" inner strength is used up coping with her child; yet she must free herself of the need to conform if she is to survive as a person who values herself and her child. She must do so in the face of a system that more often than not tells her she is a failure. This is especially true if her child's disability is behavioral or cognitive. She may even be blamed for causing it.*

---

*Interestingly, Dad is rarely the "heavy," probably because society's cultural expectations of him do not include the developmental nurturing of his children. This absolution of the father from the family's perceived deviance creates a new set of negative reactions, this time to a woman's attempt to create her wife self.

A lot—probably most—of this pain is unnecessary. It comes from forgetting what "normal" really means. That famous bell-shaped curve includes extremes at both ends; not only are they essential to define the norm, they are part of it. Put more specifically, approximately 13% of the population of the United States—some 35 million people—are handicapped to some degree. They are part of the curve and far too numerous to be considered abnormal.

With that in mind, let us go back to the creation of the self—the mystery of individual uniqueness—and that by which we measure human worth. It is important to recognize that any women's *real* (as opposed to her fantasy) image of herself as a mother is developed only in the context of real motherhood but measured against ideal concepts, the experiences of peers, and the expectations of professionals. If the pediatrician nods approval during the baby's checkup, if her baby is standing as soon (or sooner) than the neighbor's, if the milesone dates in the baby book coincide with those in her reference book, then the mother is reinforced in her new role. She feels good about the manner in which she is meeting the toughest challenge of her life and, in so doing, feels good about herself. Success breeds confidence, and confidence breeds further success.

But suppose her baby's progress lags behind the lines on the doctor's charts? Suppose he doesn't speak as soon as the neighbor's—or doesn't speak at all? If he is not developing as he should, she will at some point be forced to consider the possibility that this is her fault. It will not matter that her pediatrician or consulting specialist has diagnosed the disability as intrinsic to the child (e.g., Down's syndrome or cerebral palsy); she will question her maternal competence from conception to the present moment: I didn't eat enough fruit when I was pregnant; I should have had him without anesthesia; I let him cry too much; I left him with sitters too often. She may even decide she is being punished for some misdeed in the past.

In short, as a woman assumes what is probably the most crucial role in her adult life, her self-development in that role is going to be distorted because it is based on a distortion in feedback. Her real maternal self is created in relation to real children—not ideal ones. When one of those children reacts in an abnormal fashion because of a disability, a chain of deviance is set in motion.

Dealing with the abnormal situation can be difficult. Most of us arrive at parenthood in a sort of embryonic condition ourselves. We have been recognized as adults by society, but we are still very unformed psychologically, still very preoccupied with the business of assimilating a host of life experiences that have followed one on another in rapid succession—often overlapping—with little or no breathing space in between. We are still struggling with finding the sum of child self, adolescent self, student self, adult self, professional (or career) self, and spouse self when the new parent self comes into being. All the while most of the other selves are still evolving.

If all is going relatively well, our various selves are complementing and supplementing each other. It is when they begin to interfere with one another that we know we are in trouble. For example, when the responsibilities of the parent self overwhelm the other selves, how do we restore equilibrium? This kind of imbalance can happen in any family, but it is almost a certainty in a family with a disabled child. In either case, conflicts are to be expected.

A mother has a much better chance of what I shall term an undistorted view of disability if her handicapped child is not her firstborn. She and her husband will have had a chance to get started on the development of their parental selves in the usual fashion and, ideally, will have built up some positive self-concept in that regard. The older children will have had at least a brief period in a "normal" environment. If the handicapped child is the youngest, so much the better; the extra time and attention the child requires will not take away from—or be diminished by—the needs of a younger baby. Parents whose handicapped child is their first baby have to create their parental selves under trying circumstances; they are then likely to apply to their subsequent normal children all the apparently "abnormal" parenting skills that they were forced to develop. Perhaps the skills are better termed "extreme" (e.g., overprotections, extra caution), because all children are different and parental skills are developed differently with each child.

SOCIETAL INFLUENCES

Even if a mother accepts this view, society makes it virtually impossible for her to act on it. Girls are supposed to be prom queens and boys football stars. When she takes her disabled child to church, to the store, to the park, or even to the doctor, public reaction makes her feel obliged to explain what is "wrong" with him and to apologize—at least implicitly—for inflicting him on the normal world. Society can erode her acceptance of her child's self as he is, and therefore her acceptance of herself as a good mother to him. Eventually, unless she is an exceptionally strong person, she will come to accept society's values and expectations for her child. She will perceive both herself and her child as failures because they cannot meet those expectations. She will become angry when the physician fails to "cure," the school to "teach." She will become a service-shopper, eventually questioning her own competence when the deserved miracle doesn't occur. She may then reject this disappointing child by institutionalizing him or giving him only minimal attention, or she may devote herself entirely to him (to make up for his inadequate treatment at the hands of the professionals) and neglect her other children. Either way, her parental self has become grossly distorted.

Ironically, if she manages to hold on to the view that both she and her child are acceptable, competent, essentially normal people in a somewhat extraordinary situation, she will be challenged—by professionals, by her peers, occasionally even by herself. Acceptance of one's own competence can be terrifying, because it is the ultimate acceptance of full responsibility: no more scapegoating. At the same time, it will be her best defense against the challenges of others, challenges that come about because her acceptance has made them feel uncomfortable about themselves.

CONJUGAL RELATIONSHIPS

One of those selves that can get overlooked or distorted while everyone is focusing on the handicapped child is the wife self. Exacerbating the situation are several factors: (1) the normal jealous tension between father and children, (2) the differing expectations that fathers and mothers have of their children, and (3) the need to assign "blame" for the disaster of the handicap.

Very little needs to be said about the first; the phenomenon of a father's (particularly a first-time father) jealousy of the time and attention his wife gives the new baby has been amply recognized. We need note here only that a baby who demands even more time and attention (some of it by costly professionals) is going to force a normal parental reaction into abnormal proportions.

When it comes to differing expectations, perhaps the safest generalization is simply to state that no two parents are going to regard the same outcomes as essential for their child. Because the mother is still held to be the primary nurturer, and father the primary provider (and at least titular head of the family), their evaluations of themselves as successful parents will be based to some extent on the reflection of those roles in their children. Mother wants the child to be honest, compassionate, and happy; Dad wants financial and professional success. Mother appears more willing to be satisfied with good attempts; Father looks at actual outcomes. Of course, there are uncountable exceptions, but even when these roles are reversed, the potential for conflict exists. A child with a disability is going to have more trouble achieving traditional goals than meeting subjective ones; hence, one parent is going to suffer more acute disappointment than the other. "He's four, and he's still not talking!" "But he's trying so hard, and he communicates in other ways."

It is a very short step from that kind of exchange to a quarrel in which one parent accuses the other of being unfair to the child, and the accused counters with charges that the other is being unrealistic and refusing to face the truth. It takes more maturity than most young parents have to see the grain of truth in both positions and—more important—to realize that each is crying out from a common base of pain.

That pain is what also leads to the third divisive factor: the need to assign blame. When the disability is behavioral, that need is easily satisfied: The child's problem was clearly caused by one parent's strictness or the other's permissiveness. Even purely physical disorders are potential points of conflict, and a great deal of effort may go into proving it was her carelessness during pregnancy or his family's genes that produced the spina bifida.

If these problems are recognized as exaggerations of typical disagreements between parents, and the exaggeration itself is recognized as expected under the circumstances, they can be solved in a constructive, healthy fashion. The result will be a strengthened relationship with mutal agreement on what is best for the child. Unfortunately, it is a relationship that is hard to achieve and maintain. Instead, the conflicts described lead to more serious disagreements over management of the child and how much "abnormality" will be acceptable in the family system. If one point of view dominates, or there is a stalemate, one parent will eventually withdraw psychologically, if not physically. Either way, the practical effect is a broken marriage (the divorce rate for couples with a handicapped child is significantly higher than the national average). Even if the wife believes that she did all she could, and that *he* abandoned ship, she is still going to have to deal with the fact that she was not successful in the creation of her wife self—a commitment she made before her commitment to motherhood.

Closely related to the mother self and the wife self is the woman (adult) self. It is the sum of all the parts: child, student, professional, wife, mother, friend. Here, the presence of a handicapped child can undermine the external support system referred to earlier. A young mother's close friends generally come from three or four groups: school friends with whom she is still in touch, other mothers of young children in the neighborhood, wives of her husband's friends and professional associates, and her own professional peers if she is still working or was until the birth of her child.

When the handicapped child is still very young, these relationships can continue with little or no more external disruption than a normal child would introduce. All mothers of infants and toddlers are basically bound by their baby's needs. Even working mothers are dependent upon the availability and reliability of child care. The presence of a handicap, however, inevitably works internal modifications in these relationships—subtle fear or aversion on the part of her friends, and unconscious envy of their apparently normal lives on her part. These hidden barriers grow as the child grows. Friends may be reluctant to trade child care favors; excuses can range from the well-meaning ("I just would be afraid to take that responsibility. I think the way you manage is wonderful!") to the unconsciously cruel ("I'd love to take David for the afternoon, but he makes my kids nervous"). The mother's envy of her friends grows; they have freedom; she's stuck at first base. The gulf widens when the children reach school age. The handicapped child may have to attend a private school with shorter hours and/or no transportation; so when her peers go back to work or become active in community affairs, she is still tied down. As the children reach the age when they no longer need sitters, their parents regain social independence; *she* will probably never have it. Spontaneous, spur-of-the-moment activities are out of the question, even when her offspring reaches adulthood. As the child ages, the situation can become more deviant until there is virtually no commonality between her life and those of her friends.

SOLUTIONS

There are two possible solutions: total isolation from everyone except family (sometimes even from family—siblings of handicapped children have been known to leave home early, and retarded persons are often excluded from family events such as weddings) or total absorption into the subculture of the handicapped. In the latter case, the parents (singly or together) join an organization devoted to their child's disability. They make new friends with other parents and become totally caught up in the "cause." It is still an isolated existence, but it can be personally reinforcing. In fact, it may be the only concretely beneficial thing they can ever do for their child. Furthermore, it can mean psychological survival for a woman who—besides losing the social support of her "normal" friends—has been deprived of peer standards by which to assess herself as a woman. The supermom with three normal kids, who bakes her own bread, holds a full-time job, and chairs the local political club has no relevance for her; she must find other, appropriate models by which to measure herself, other friends whose commonality of experience and need will bind her to them and them to her.

If she can find this type of accepting environment, she can grow because of her child's disability, not in spite of it. The disability will be an accepted, legitimate part of the child's self, and the child will be a positive part of the mother's self-image. When this happens, both she and her child will be free to realize their individual goals without undue concern for society's ingrained norms.

Unfortunately, the mother of a handicapped child is still very likely to be thwarted by the "helping" professions. The dominance of the medical model with its orientation toward curing (in child psychiatry, "rescuing") the child perpetuates reliance on an inappropriate norm. Her grief at her child's disability is appropriate—and permanent—and must be accepted as such. Her efforts to alleviate the effects of the impairment are usually healthy and not indications of denial; her desire to have part of her life purely for herself is positive selfishness, not escapism. Until professionals accept these concepts in practice as well as in theory, they will be of no more help to mothers of handicapped children than were the toy makers who produced the perfect dolls of her childhood.

Chapter 8

Mothers of the Retarded

Norman R. Bernstein

Almost all mothers fear a defective child. Today such fears are amplified by the news of possible causes of mental retardation, concern about food additives, phenylketonuria, radiation hazards, and fetal alcohol syndrome, as well as by widely disseminated media reports on genetic counseling, Down's syndrome, and the hazards of nitrites, ordinary medications, and dietary patterns. Much unassimilated information contributes to the vague apprehension that terrible things can happen to a fetus. Folk tales about sex during the final stages of pregnancy and about youthful indiscretions still cause people to become fearful about producing retarded children. In addition, some individuals may worry about having relatives who are intellectually handicapped or who had abnormal births. Brewer and Kakalik (1979) estimate that currently in the United States there are nearly 3 million retarded youths age 21 or younger.

The burden of raising retarded children falls most heavily on the mother, even if the father is enlightened, loving, and helpful. From the time in pregnancy when there is a risk of rubella or other viral infections, when the doctors caution about smoking and alcohol intake, when amniocentesis may be suggested, the mother may become frightened about what is growing within her in a way that cannot be experienced by men. A family history of fetal wastage, congenital anomalies, childhood psychosis, or other similar aberrations adds to the woman's terror. At the infant's birth, physicians may recognize multiple handicaps, and the mother may be asked not to see her child immediately because of emergency procedures. Severe types of mental retardation can be manifested by microcephaly and anencephaly. Congenital disor-

Norman R. Bernstein • Department of Psychiatry, Harvard Medical School, Cambridge, Massachusetts 02140.

ders such as cerebral palsy can be diagnosed at birth. In addition to the direct diagnosis of handicaps, the mother may be told that the doctor is worried that the child has jaundice or does not suck or move vigorously. Some mothers worry when their newborns are sluggish and sleepy, although the doctor has not suggested that anything is wrong. This early pattern of sleeping and waking relates to the amount of anesthesia that has been given as well as to the baby's constitutional endowment or temperament, an area that has been extensively studied by Thomas and Chess (1968).

These authors identified specific characteristics to judge children's temperament. The child's activity level is defined by the frequency and speed of movement, whether wiggling in the bath or crib in early infancy, or crawling, walking, and running later. The child's rhythmicity is defined according to its biological regularity as seen in such functions as the sleep–waking cycle and the timing of hunger and defecation. Approach-withdrawal is the child's immediate reaction (acceptance or rejection) to a new experience, such as a bed, a place, a person, or a schedule.

The child's adaptability to a new experience or schedule is measured by the amount of time (short, moderate, or long) the child requires to make the transition. Threshold is the minimum strength of the child's reaction. Intensity is the energy expended in expressing a mood without regard to the nature of the mood itself. Mood is defined as the predominance of positive mood during waking hours as opposed to neutral or negative mood. Distractibility refers to the ease with which the child's attention is drawn from an ongoing activity by a peripheral stimulus and directed toward a new one. Attention span refers to the child's ability to concentrate without interruption, such as gazing at a moving object, and persistence refers to continuous uninterrupted activity toward the completion of a task.

Chess and co-workers point out that these qualities can be altered by experience but tend to derive from innate sources. When a child who is retarded seems to have a low activity level and to be rhythmic, slightly withdrawn, and pleasant in mood, a parent may often feel that the child is a "lazy baby" or an "easy baby" and nothing is wrong organically. Coexisting with the tremendous apprehension of many mothers is a great capacity to deny signs of retardation. The mother may not be bothered by the child's inability to sit, walk, or talk on time and may even be reassured by a sanguine pediatrician that the child will develop slowly. For this reason, the diagnosis of mental retardation is likely to be made at the time of a child's school entry, when developmental assessments and educational evaluation may uncover developmental lags that the parents have disavowed.

Of the 3% of the population diagnosed as mentally retarded, about

85% are mildly retarded; that is, they have an IQ between 60 and 70. Hence, milder forms of retardation predominate and diagnostic error is not uncommon, particularly when coupled with parents' denial. Parents' attitudes toward retardation reflect their values. Some parents state, "We'd rather have a child with psychiatric problems that can be treated than a child who is permanently retarded."

Solnit and Stark (1963) report: "Parenthood for most couples is a crisis situation even when their child is born healthy. When a defective child is born, the crisis is magnified. The fears of the mother have come true; in place of a wished for, fantasized child, the mother reacts to the loss of her hopes and fantasies as if the child had suddenly died and she grieves and mourns its loss." Solnit and Stark wrote that this characteristic response accompanies the loss of a valued object, be it a person, possession, job, status, home country, part of the body, or ideal. The birth of a retarded child, however, is surrounded by a complicating cluster of phenomena.

The constellation of hopes that a mother has for a male or female baby are both conscious and unconscious, simple and intricate, immediate and long-term. In each of these categories the mother's emotions shift toward wounding, bereavement, and mortification when the child is said to be deficient (Bernstein, 1970). In every society mental retardation is a handicap—it hinders the individual's functioning and diminishes the individual's opportunities for a happy and fulfilling life (Jackson, 1974). Olshansky (1966) writes that mental retardation is unaesthetic. It is not an attractive or poetic disease. Kanner (1962) points out that society has been overwhelmingly negative about the retarded.

Most workers in this field are aware that the mother's reaction to the child's disability may influence the child's development as much as, if not more than, the disability itself. Although fathers react initially to the mother's grief, they generally express more thoughts about long-term outcomes of retardation, losing their hopes for a gratifying relationship to a grown son or daughter. Mothers tend to focus on the more immediate tragedy, but both parents are likely to have a surge of guilt derived from a general feeling that they have done something for which they are being punished. Such guilt occurs among educated and sophisticated parents as readily as it does among medically uninformed parents and is a complex derivative of personality structure. Mothers may also feel they have failed their husbands by producing a defective child.

Some mothers are more suffused with shame, a sense that their child's defectiveness will stigmatize them among their relatives, in-laws, and friends. This sense of public stigma affects all mothers who want a beautiful child to enhance their own self-esteem. They begin to feel that the handicapped child is an unavoidable burden on their lives (Voisey,

1975). The retarded child and its reverberations may be a severely disruptive influence on the family, affecting the development of other children and the pattern of relationships between the mother and father.

DECLARING THE DIAGNOSIS

There are many problems concerning who should tell the family (the pediatrician, the obstetrician, a pediatric neurologist, a teacher, or a psychologist), how the family should be told, how many times they should be told, and whether the diagnosis is understood and accepted. Some cannot accept that the child is retarded; they focus instead on a minor point the doctor has raised and thereby avoid the bad news. This reaction may be linked to the doctor's delivery of the information; he or she may identify with the mother, fail to speak clearly, and hedge the diagnosis with euphemisms. The pediatrician who has been through several illnesses with a mother and her other children is more likely to be able to form an alliance during a crisis.

In our transient society, however, it is unlikely that the person telling the mother will know her very well. Too often experts in genetic counseling begin to give the mother information about further pregnancies before the mother has had a few months to absorb what has happened to her. When parents hear that their child is defective, they may be devastated by a barrage of genetic statistics about further risks to other children they may conceive (Goshen, 1964; Kanner, 1962).

Today's technology enhances the ability of neonatologists to "salvage" premature infants of body weights under 1,000 grams; in fact, infants as small as 500 grams may be saved. The 1,000-gram neonate has a 25% chance of suffering brain insult and retardation; for the 500-gram infant, such chances increase to almost 50%. These scientific advances bring with them major moral issues and emotional traumas for parents (Henig, 1981).

PATTERNS OF MOTHERS AND FAMILIES

There are many myths about how parents manage the birth of a retarded child. Attempts to describe family types that handle retarded children are not adequately documented (Deutch, 1945). Tizard (1964) notes that it is often said that mothers in poor families have a greater tolerance for mentally retarded children. However, he says no evidence exists to substantiate this theory. Women who are extremely concerned about the appearance and performance of their children will probably have a particularly difficult time, but all parents are shocked and mortified. Strong religious faith helps parents to cope. Religiously devout parents consider the retarded child to be a special blessing; the child provides them with challenges that will improve them spiritually.

Nevertheless, parents who write some of the more dramatic and positive articles may privately be much more negative and disconcerted about their situation (Hart, 1970). The strengths of the family that enable them to deal with a retarded child are often not immediately discernible. Unless a woman has grown up with a retarded sibling, she is not likely to be familiar with the issues and problems involved, even though retardation is a relatively common condition, afflicting 3% of the population. Our society has tended to camouflage the retarded, relegating them to a different world of the handicapped that is hidden from public attention. Bias against the retarded resembles bias against the poor minorities and the chronically ill and leads to the social theory that all those who fall into these categories have a greater tolerance for boring work than does the general public. Another central theme is that there is no escape from retardation. The defect is permanent, the problems endure, and these facts add to the sense of hopelessness of so many mothers.

The preoccupations of obsessional women may take the form of reading everything available on retardation and organizing rituals of child care. For some women who feel most gratified caring for a young infant, the prolonged dependency of the retarded child may provide a longer caretaking period of special pleasure and identification with the helplessness of the child. Usually the woman's sense of personhood, confidence, and completeness is assailed. Her reproductive capacities appear impaired, however logically she may disavow this judgment. For some women, their previous psychopathology may be irrelevant; for example, a highly neurotic woman can put aside her phobias, hypochondriasis, moodiness, and thin-skinned attitudes to meet the challenge of a serious problem. Although the majority of parents of retarded children do not collapse, they show signs of chronic stress, some constriction of their life-styles, and greater focus on the needs of the impaired child. Sources of help may lie within a larger extended family network as well as in community medical and mental health services.

SIBLINGS

A handicapped child may become the negative center of home life. Mothers may demand that siblings help with diapering and baby-sitting, take the retarded child for walks or to the movies, and include him or her in games. The most exquisite agonies may be felt when parents insist that their normal adolescent children take the mentally handicapped child to social events. The following vignettes are derived from the author's clinical and teaching experience.

One physician described growing up in a middle-class home with a moderately retarded sister. When he was 8 or 9 years old, he felt ashamed when he was seen with her. He was kind at home, but when he watched her fumble in the supermarket he became irritable with her. He felt that her stigma as "retarded" contaminated him. A compliant child, he did what his mother wanted and included his sister in many activities. At age 12 he was greatly embarrassed when she sat on the sidelines while he played sandlot baseball. Later, he feared his dates would learn too soon that he had a mentally deficient sister at home. Occasionally he wished she would be sent away or that she would simply die. These fantasies were always followed by surges of guilt and new efforts to help out with his sister.

When he took psychology and child psychiatry courses in college and medical school, his sense of shame was blended with new knowledge about cognitive handicaps. Intellectualizing helped him distance himself from the phenomenon of mental handicap, and he never wanted to work with the retarded professionally. He said he had long struggled to keep his family problem a secret, although he continued to do his duty, giving medical advice and arranging a trust fund for his sister's care in later life. When he married, he did not want his wife to have his sister visit or have his own normal children associate with his sister.

Another young man from a poor family in London was a juvenile delinquent; he got into many violent fights, railed at policemen, broke into warehouses, and had numerous scrapes with the law. When he was in his 20s, working regularly as a maintenance man and electrician, his retarded sister was released from a school for the retarded. The local clinic arranged for her to live alone and advised her to use contraceptives. She got pregnant and had an abortion. Her brother took over responsibility for her, insisting that she go back to her residential setting in a church home. He visited her weekly, transported her home for visits, and collaborated with his parents on family parties for Christmas and Easter. Anyone who looked askance at his sister's awkward social behavior could provoke him to violence. "I'd cosh a guy," the young man said, "but I'd never use a shooter." He treated her with the same strictness and devotion with which he treated a huge German shepherd he had trained. He righteously refused to permit her any sexual experience, although he was quite promiscuous himself.

The domestic care of a handicapped child is still likely to be assumed primarily by the child's sisters. Some mothers of the retarded invoke sympathy for themselves, some simply demand that their daughters help out, while others try to spare their daughters some of the stigma. One young woman who had a retarded brother recalled the ambivalent attitudes of her family while she was growing up in the

Midwest. The home milieu felt dark and cold. Her father said all the correct things but avoided his retarded son as much as possible; her mother was unreliable and irascible, and would abruptly shunt her son's care over to the younger sister. The sister felt her friends were not welcome in the home.

Another young women served as a rescuer in emergency situations. Her 21-year-old brother lived at home with their parents. He had held a job loading and unloading trucks at a supermarket but lost the job when the market went bankrupt. While he was growing up, his mother had dutifully brought him for special schooling and had not been troubled by his interest in girls or his solitary masturbation. After he lost his job, he began to wander in the streets of their small town and was arrested after following some young girls. His mother was paralyzed with embarrassment, contrition, and rage at her son; she refused to go to the police station or the mental retardation clinic to which he was referred. Instead, his married sister brought him to the clinic and made all the arrangements for him, in order to spare her mother. The sister was firmly opposed to taking him into her home, however, even on a respite basis.

Schwartz (1975) has studied the status of the family of the retarded and reports that socioeconomic status is a major influence. For the affluent family, the birth of a retarded child is a crisis of *ends;* the mother can no longer think of the child's college or professional careers, marriage, or grandchildren. The child will be unable to fulfill her hopes or bear the torch of her ambitions to the next generation. For the poor family, the crisis is one of *means.* The family must devote a great deal of energy to finding ways of getting the child to the clinic, the special class, and the specialists.

Klaus and Kennell (1970) suggest that a lack of early physical contact may retard the attachment between a mother and her child and in turn may cause the mother to spend less time fondling and looking and smiling at her baby. This observation relates to the skewed interactional patterns described by Goldfarb (1961), who has noted that a mother does not react as well to the deviant child who is not emitting responsive signals as she would to normal offspring. Thus, the child becomes puzzled and emits even more distorted responses, which sets up an unsatisfactory, vicious cycle.

CHILD ABUSE

Some of the violence perpetrated against children may be linked to the desperation of mothers with retarded children. The retarded child may become the special target for the overburdened, impoverished, and isolated mother, or such a mother may be unable to protect the child from an abusing father (Brandewein, 1973).

CASE 1. Mrs. P was a 34-year-old suburban housewife. Her husband, an emotionally detached scientist, spent all of his spare time working at the computer terminal in the cellar of their Tudor house. Mrs. P had an austere, deprived upbringing in New England. When she became agitated and despairing, she slapped her 2½-year-old retarded child. At these times, she never struck her other normal child, however. Mrs. P was a chronically dissatisfied woman whose anger toward her husband was partly displaced on her retarded child. Although she sought psychiatric help several times, she always left the session in a rage because she felt the doctors would not do enough for her.

Some mothers remain hopeful, regardless of what they have been told by professionals. They see progress in their children; they have read of scientific advances. Dietary measures to prevent or ameliorate phenylketonuria are frequently cited in reports as an example of a clear and often effective method of intervention. Similarly, the use of the thyroid to combat cretinism gives some parents hope that scientific breakthroughs will cure their children. Some also hope retardation will be rediagnosed as a metabolic imbalance that is curable.

CAUSES AND CRUSADES

Some years ago Wolfensburger (1967) reported the rage of parents toward the professionals who care for their retarded children. Most parents of the retarded do not feel they have been well served by teachers, pediatricians, neurologists, psychiatrists, social workers, or psychologists. Professionals entering the field of retardation are warned about the wrath of parents. This wrath is triggered by the parents' feeling that they have been wronged by life as well as by the inadequacy of the services available for the parents and the insensitivities of many of the caretaking professionals.

Some mothers who become involved in organizations for the retarded find a much-needed outlet for their feelings of despair. They meet other parents who also experience the "chronic sorrow" that Olshansky (1966) delineated—a psychological state that differs from the loss of a child through death. It combines a loss of the image and hopes surrounding a normal child with the continuing challenges the retarded child produces. This chronic sorrow should be treated by psychotherapists as a neurotic conflict that can be resolved. It is a heavy, intractable reality. Thus, parents who fight the state department of mental health or campaign for new legislation and funding can be improving the quality of life for the mentally retarded as well as sublimating their own personal bitterness.

THE LONG-TERM CONSEQUENCES

The financial consequences of retardation are enormous. The state or the family must provide special support systems to help the retarded function. While parents occasionally joke that by having a retarded child they are spared the costs of college education, over a lifetime the costs of caring for a mentally retarded child are much greater than those for a normal child.

The mothers of the retarded must remain on guard to protect their children and avoid embarrassing encounters. They must fend off hurtful bystanders and deal with their own attitudes about their impaired children. Rarely are they totally without some rejecting impulses of their own. Stone (1948) has pointed out that parents feel guilty about their tendency to reject the retarded child; he notes that the defective child often quite consciously becomes the pawn in a battle between marital partners, a situation illustrated by the following case.

CASE 2. Mrs. K married at age 22. Her first child was a handicapped infant with a cleft palate, a harelip, lower-limb paralysis, and gross mental retardation. Mrs. K's husband was an energetic business executive who traveled a great deal. Mrs. K had prided herself on her appearance and the perfection of her home; in many ways she was a conventional wife who felt very comfortable depending on, and being cared for by, her husband. Her first words after the delivery, when she had seen the child and spoke to her husband, were "I've given you a bad baby."

From that time on, the character of her life changed, and her relationship with her husband was altered and diluted. Mrs. K began to focus all of her activities on the child, paying much less attention to, and showing little sexual interest in, her husband. The child was maintained at home for 14 years, even though he never progressed beyond the mental age of a 5-month-old infant. A great deal of time and money was spent taking him to specialists. Mr. K withdrew more and more into his work and into flying lessons, which had a quality of reckless desperation; Mrs. K quartered her mother nearby to help care for the child and then moved her mother into the house, which further alienated her husband. Her own long-standing feelings of dependency and inadequacy were intensified by this catastrophic event. The situation persisted while the child lived at home; by the time he was a teenager and had been moved to an institution, the marriage seemed irreparably damaged.

Their second child was a normal girl, who felt that too much attention was paid to her brother because of his handicap. She was teased in the neighborhood as the sister of a "retard" and struggled for years to distance herself from feeling contaminated by his defect. She went to college, married, and left home, bearing a chronic animosity toward both of her parents: She resented her father for permitting an undue focus on her handicapped brother, and she resented her mother for not being emotionally available.

At age 26 the retarded son died of pulmonary infection. The parents took steps toward separation and divorce. Mrs. K felt that she had poured all of her vital energies into caring for her retarded son, but when he died she felt that she had to take over the care of her own aging mother, who was now sickly. Mr. K felt that he could not tolerate this withdrawal of attention and support. Mrs. K went for counseling with her husband before and after their separation. She opened a boutique and partially recovered from her despair. Essentially she tried to resume her personal development, arrested since adolescence. Mr. K sought out a woman who was devoted in her care of him to make up for what he felt he had lacked.

THE REALITIES OF CARING FOR A RETARDATE

One hears about parents who could not get sitters for their retarded 25-year-olds and who felt chained to them. Failure to gain respite from a normal child is bothersome enough to parents, but the endless dependency of a mentally defective child can be dreadful. Parents have great fears about the sexuality of their retarded sons and daughters. They have heard stories about young girls being lured into prostitution, and certainly it is difficult to cope with a retarded adolescent girl who has strong sexual feelings that she wants to express. One father said, "Judy has the mind of a six-year-old but the body of an eighteen-year-old." Parents' own guilt about sexuality recrudesces when they confront these issues. Stories about aggressive child molesters who are retarded plague parents.

The issue of sex education for the retarded is rife with conflicts. Modern institutions have attempted to socialize the retarded by allowing them to share time with the opposite sex. Frequently, staff members have become outraged over the sex play that goes on—homosexual, heterosexual, and autoerotic. Parents who are fairly sophisticated about their own sexuality or about that of normal children are sometimes desperate with guilt and anxiety when facing their retarded children's sexuality. The defective is sexually stimulated by magazines, newspapers, television, and films but is taught that he or she is in a "different" category in terms of sexuality. Doctors and counselors frequently convey their own ambivalence by simultaneously advocating free expression, acceptance, and a primitive desire to suppress sexuality in the retarded. Thus, parents have problems getting clear messages. Reliable, permanent communication channels remain a high priority for the parents of the retarded (Coughlin, 1941).

CASE 3. Mrs. L was a 55-year-old wife of a prosperous lawyer. She had five children, among whom was Jane, their fourth child, a 27-year-old daughter with an IQ of 56. Jane was discharged from a reputable school for the retarded with good self-care skills. When she returned to live with her parents, they had moved from their suburban home to downtown Chicago, within easy walking distance of the pornography and prostitution district. Jane wandered in this area and found men with whom she would have sex. She delighted in the attention, the erotic experience, and the overwhelming reaction of her distraught parents.

Her father said he would pay to send Jane away to another school, but he was not active in the decision making. Her mother had been reluctant to have a child at home again after all of them had been away for several years, especially at a time when she was focusing on country clubs, museum boards, and her own cultural development. Although another daughter's hippy phase and open promiscuity had outraged Mrs. L's religious and moral sensibilities, she had hoped that the daughter knew "what she was doing." She could not harbor the same hope for Jane, however; eventually Jane's promiscuity became extremely unsettling to her mother and led to her return to an institutional setting.

The family must deal with the social stigma of having a retarded child. The mother feels this stigma when she takes her Mongoloid infant to the supermarket, when she takes her child to special classes, when she stands guard over her child socially. Despite the emphasis on Special Olympics, work programs, and psychotherapy reports on the retarded, retarded children have traditionally been taught to be passive. Naturally, passive children will pose fewer problems for their parents (Zola, 1982). Thus, parents may feel that passivity helps to minimize stigma.

Who Endures

Most parents survive, but they do not always develop the tolerance and depth of feeling that some authorities predict. Many become bitter, suspicious, or exhausted. One feature that seems to be decisive is physical vigor. Mothers need patience and energy to toilet-train a retarded child at age 7 or 8, to keep trying to indoctrinate a child who does not seem to comprehend, and to continue guarding a child who does not socialize well.

Ninety-five percent of the retarded live in the community. Although roughly 3% of all children are diagnosed as being retarded, when we try to follow up retarded children in adult life, we find that two-thirds of them have disappeared into the general population. If they are not in trouble with the draft board or the Internal Revenue Service, we can find only 1% of the retarded in the adult population. Thus, in spite of the parents' disappointments, a great many of the retarded learn to function in the community. We do not have good data on how the retarded age, what their illness statistics are, or how they relate to their families.

However, an enormous amount of anecdotal information indicates that some of the mothers' burden is shifted to the community or is borne by others outside the family—friends, spouses, and lovers of these retarded adults, the vast majority of whom are mildly retarded.

BEING REALISTIC AND MAINTAINING HOPE

We never expect mothers of normal children to be realistic. We expect them to be benignly and madly happy about their unique and talented offspring. Onlookers take delight in this parental joy. The pleasure of parenthood is related, in part, to the legitimate opportunity to indulge in the most unrealistic hopes and fantasies of one's child. The mother of a retarded child, however, is expected to be realistic—realistic about doctor's appointments, about the lack of efficacious treatment, about what her child can do, and about how the child will behave in the midst of the most conflicted and frightening reports from society. Yet, over the long run, most parents manage to deal with the family realignment caused by the birth of a retarded child and with the child's limitations. Generally families become more integrated: Siblings bear some of the responsibility, and the parents' ambivalence only occasionally interferes with the management of the retarded child.

Mothers of the mentally handicapped must plan for their children beyond maturity and after their own deaths. They will not receive help from these children in later life. If possible, they should set up trust funds to help in the care of these children. They should also attempt to negotiate with their other children to assume the roles of conservator, trustee, and caretaker.

Mothers of the retarded have not been treated fairly. Departments of mental health and mental retardation continue to combine, separate, and recombine as funds diminish; retardation services generally suffer the most. The staffs of these organizations also are divided between the mental health and the mental retardation fields, and mental health staff often don't want to work with retardates. Too often the mother of a retarded child is treated as if she were neurotic, as if therapy could alter an unfortunate reality. In fact, her chronic sorrow, suspiciousness, and fatigue are the products of a relentless problem and not that of unconscious conflict (Jakab, 1982).

Some mothers can obtain parental gratification from their other children. One mother of two severely retarded children had two normal daughters who gave her great pleasure. In middle life she went to social work school and then cared for burned children, feeling they were different enough from the retarded to permit her some distance while allowing her to apply her own experience in a socially helpful way.

In our society, mothering a defective child does not provide the kind of self-enhancing developmental experience that normal childrearing produces (Szymanski & Tanguay, 1980). Generally it provides only a sense of a loss, which alters the mother's personality by strengthening her adaptive defenses. Eventually these defenses harden into a pattern of merely trying to survive under the strain of permanent vigilance over the retarded child.

REFERENCES

Bernstein, N. (1970). *Diminished people*. Boston: Little, Brown.

Brandewein, H. (1973). The battered child: A definite and significant factor in mental retardation, *Mental Retardation, 11*(5), 50–51.

Brewer, G., & Kakalik, J. (1979). *Handicapped children: Strategies for improving services.* New York: McGraw-Hill.

Coughlin, E. W. (1941). Some parental attitudes toward handicapped children. *Child, 6,* 41–45.

Deutch, H. (1945). *The psychology of women, II: Motherhood.* New York: Grune & Stratton.

Goldfarb, W. (1961). *Childhood Schizophrenia.* Cambridge, MA: Harvard University Press.

Goshen, C. E. (1964). Mental retardation and neurotic maternal attitudes. *Archives of General Psychiatry, 9,* 168–174.

Hart, N. (1970). Frequently expressed feelings and reactions of parents toward their retarded children. In N. R. Bernstein (Ed.), *Diminished people.* Boston: Little, Brown.

Henig, R. (1981). Now we must face the dark side of the premie miracle. *Chicago Tribune,* March 29, Section 12, p. 1.

Jackson, P. (1974). Chronic grief. *American Journal of Nursing, 74,* 1289–1291.

Jakab, I. (Ed.). (1982). *Mental retardation.* New York: Karger.

Kanner, L. (1962). *A history of the care and study of the mentally retarded.* Springfield, IL: Charles C Thomas.

Klaus, M., & Kennell, J. (1970). Mothers separated from their newborn infants. *Pediatric Clinics of North America, 17*(4), 1015–1037.

Olshansky, S. (1966). Parent responses to a mentally defective child. *Mental Retardation, 4,* 21–23.

Schwartz, C. (1970). Strategies and tactics of mothers of mentally retarded children for dealing with the medical care system. Chap. 5, pp. 73–106, in *Diminished people,* ed. N. Bernstein. Boston: Little, Brown.

Solnit, A., & Stark, M. (1963). Mourning and the birth of a defective child. *Psychoanalytic Study of the Child, 16,* 523–537.

Stone, M. (1948). Parental attitudes to retardation. *American Journal of Mental Deficiency, 53,* 363–372.

Szymanski, L., & Tanguay, P. (1980). *Emotional disorders of mentally retarded persons: Assessment, treatments and consultation.* Baltimore: University Park Press.

Thomas, A., & Chess, S. (1968). *Temperament and behavior disorders in children.* New York: New York University Press.

Tizard, J. (1964). *Community services for the mentally handicapped.* New York: Oxford University Press.

Voisey, M. (1975). *A constant burden.* London: Routledge & Kegan Paul.

Wolfensburger, W. (1967). Counseling parents of the retarded. In A. A. Baumeister (Ed.), *Mental retardation: Appraisal, education and rehabilitation.* Chicago: Aldine.

Zola, I. (1982). *Missing pieces.* Philadelphia: Temple University Press.

PART IV

Women with Extraordinary Problems

Chapter 9

On Becoming Empowered

Peggy Dulany

Empowerment is another term for finding one's own voice. In order to speak, we must know what we want to say; in order to be heard, we must dare to speak. Coming to know and coming to dare, being empowered, are all part of a complicated process. Part of that process happens through the biological course of growing up. Another part is affected by the reception we find in this world of ours.

In the ideal democracy everyone has the opportunity to find his or her voice and to use it with equal force. In reality, circumstances militate against such equality. Imbalances, born of historical injustices, perpetuate themselves and harden into patterns. Those who feel historically as well as individually mute need even greater courage to gain a sense of their own power; they have to achieve not only a sense of power but the actual power as well. Usually, empowerment occurs through contact with others who are empowered, who have found their voices and who speak clearly and loudly, rather than dictate. It happens when people who have been muted and gagged for generations are offered the opportunity to mumble and cry, and finally to speak, shout, and sing out.

Empowerment also suggests helping others find the knowledge and courage to speak with their own voice. Collective empowerment is social change, because when enough people enunciate their beliefs in unison, they will be heard and society will respond.

It is not useful to speak about empowering large groups of people, however, without first finding clarity within ourselves. Some suggestions are offered as possible avenues for becoming empowered.

Peggy Dulany • The Synergos Institute, New York, New York 10028.

EMPOWERMENT VIA WORK-RELATED EXPERIENCES

The variety of internal and external circumstances that affect growth toward empowerment was the focus of two research studies in which I was engaged—one in 1964, another in 1974. The objectivity and the replicability of either the design or the execution of these studies are open to debate. They were probably more meaningful to the author in clarifying a sense of self and thinking about this process than in advancing the science of human psychology.

Between 1965 and 1969, summers and part of one winter were spent on doing anthropological fieldwork in *favelas,* or squatter settlements, in Rio de Janeiro, Brazil. Most of the people living there had come from rural settings throughout Brazil. Arriving in Rio, they had to learn to cope with new experiences that must have been mind-boggling. Mostly illiterate, they had to learn to navigate a giant city full of unfamiliar signs, with a transit system as complex as that of any major city in the world. Many of the migrants, having only worked as field laborers, had to adjust to the notions of bureaucracy, timetables, and corruption. In Rio, they entered a world saturated with television, which was novel not only in its technology but also for its portrayal of middle-class values and life-styles. Previously they knew no one more different from themselves than the parish priest, who might have come from another village, or the local landowner, who might have attended the state university; every day in Rio they were faced with a wide range of people from all over the country. They found themselves in a class and color system that was both defined and subtle, a pecking order that was as rigid as it was unspoken.

I became preoccupied with discovering the mechanisms that helped the survivors adapt to this new world. Why did others fail to adapt—those who went crazy, or couldn't hold a job, or went back to the roça, as the interior was called? Conversations with many people and a trip to the interior with the host family provoked speculations that two factors were crucial to successful adaptation to this new life: First, some previous experience, no matter how different from that of city life, seemed to lend a perspective that made it easier to cope with the novelty of the city. Second, relatives or fellow villagers who had migrated to the same *favela* provided an external support system; such social or religious associations offered the migrants companionship and tension relief.

After college, circumstances made it impractical to continue the research in Brazil. That research experience stimulated insight into some larger social phenomena that affect people's capacity to cope and adapt; however, it had not promoted insight into the complex interaction of internal and external factors that form our personalities. These issues were addressed during my graduate work experience (in psychology and education) and that of directing an alternative high school for dropout students.

The experience with students whose failure in school was a symptom of a far greater sense of failure in life confirmed the concepts that had been learned in developmental psychology: The natural growth process can be severely stunted or warped when the external environment does not nurture it. A stable home environment with loving parents, appropriate exposure to challenging experiences, and positive reinforcement for meeting those challenges encourage development and foster openness to further growth. But societal factors such as racism, sexism, and classism, unstable home bases, lack of opportunity for exposure to new experiences, or too much exposure with too little support can prevent adolescents from finding their own voices.

Many of the adolescents in the program had led traumatic and difficult lives since childhood; not surprisingly, they were reluctant to take any risks that might further confirm their already powerful sense of failure. The school failure that had led to their dropping out was often precipitated by their refusal to risk trying. And that refusal was a mechanism for preventing further erosion of self-esteem after so many other apparent failures—at home, where parents who were unable to set consistent limits blamed them for not obeying sometimes arbitrary rules, and on the street, where they were often in trouble with the law.

Some of these students considered returning to school in the program, a preferable alternative to jail; for others, attendance in the program revealed their residual hope that one more try would not automatically end in failure. The courage of this latter group grew out of a strong human need to feel competent. Only when society shuts young people out of respectable pursuits do they try to excel in less acceptable activities. As a successful thief, or thug, or hooker, or dealer, they would at least earn the admiration of peers who had also been excluded by society.

How can such adolescents be encouraged to risk expressing not only their sorrow and rage, but their ideas and aspirations? The school staff found that students had to feel safe from further failure before they were willing to try again. It was necessary to construct an atmosphere that was predictable, to set limits consistently, and to be caring so that the students could believe the staff both wanted them to succeed and thought they could. Then, for each individual, staff sought out any existing areas of competence—whether that was in friendship, art, sports, work, or some aspect of academic learning—and began building further confidence on that foundation. The school became a safe haven where students could take small risks, just as the support of the hometown neighbors makes it possible for new migrants to the *favela* to cope with city life.

A supportive environment that programmed success into the pursuit of competence allowed these fragile young people to construct a foundation of self-esteem on which to build bridges to other areas of endeavor. For instance, three boys felt comfortable only in their friendship with each other and their skill in stealing cars. In their English class, however, they felt uncomfortable and inept. For months they disrupted the class with raucous comparisons of their exploits. I finally made a deal with them: They could talk only about the exploits they had written down. This bargain led to highly imaginative and amusing stories—with titles like "Charlie the Himalayan Monk" or "Fred the Speed-Freak Monster"—in which the boys tried to surpass each other with exaggerations of outlandish acts.

After a few weeks, the boys were comfortable with writing; they were no longer terrified of being mocked or punished for having a fourth-grade spelling ability in the tenth grade. They began to ask me or each other how to spell different words. More traditional grammar and spelling lessons were interspersed into their less orthodox, but certainly more creative, efforts at expression.

Once the students felt safe in the school environment, they would try to strengthen their competence in other skills. This process of risking a new experience, integrating the lesson into one's sense of self, and then opening up to further new experiences represents a universal process of growth. By testing our metaphorical voice in different rooms, at different pitches, and with varying degrees of loudness and intensity, we begin to determine the range that rings true. Thus, we learn to project with the sweetest sound.

BECOMING EMPOWERED WITHIN ONE'S FAMILY

Growing up as a member of the Rockefeller family is a unique experience in some ways. Therefore, my examples of finding my own voice may seem irrelevant to the experiences of many others. However, I am convinced that the process of finding one's own voice is common to us all.

During the summer of 1967, I returned to Rio for the third time. Instead of living with the wealthy friends of my family and commuting daily to the *favela*, I decided to live in a *favela* called Jacarezinho with a family I had come to know. This family and a few other people in the *favela* knew I was a Rockefeller; they were nonplussed by my background, however, perhaps because it seemed so implausible.

In contrast, my decision to live in a *favela* decidedly upset the Braza (a pseudonym) family with whom I had previously lived. The father was angry that I would choose such a site over his lovely house. He was fearful for my safety, and yet awed by my apparent craziness. At a cocktail party he could not resist telling the story to some of his friends, including the owner of the biggest gossip magazine in Brazil.

I did not realize anything was amiss until one day when I was doing an interview in the *favela*. A fellow researcher, the wife of our team leader, burst into the house. She called me aside and informed me that a *Jornal Do Brasil* truck was making its way up the only road wide enough to accommodate a vehicle. The truck was blaring over its loudspeaker that the magazine would pay for any information about the Rockefeller who was working in the *favela*. She told me I had to get out of there as soon as possible and never come back or I would ruin the research study.

In shock, I left quickly and jumped on the first bus back to Jacarezinho. The family with whom I was living locked me in a room as soon as I arrived. They gave me a solution of sugar and water to calm me down and told me that there had been reporters on the roofs of the surrounding houses all afternoon, watching for my return. Just as I had arrived, the reporters had left for a moment to make a phone call at the police station. Thus, they were unaware of my return. As darkness approached, the reporters' fears of the *favela* overcame their desire to get the story, and they retreated.

I was in such a state of panic that my only thought was to leave the city. I had been planning to visit the state of Bahia at some point during the summer; a friend and I decided we might as well do it then. Fearing that by the next day the bus station, train terminal, port, and airport would all be staked out by reporters, we took an overnight bus to São Paulo, 250 miles to the south, and caught another bus the next morning, retracing our steps 1,000 miles north. The entire trip lasted 56 hours!

This experience would be unnerving for any 19-year-old, but what caused my disproportionate panic? In the *favela*, for the first time in my life, I had been able to feel absolutely comfortable with a group of people—both my co-workers and the family with whom I was living. My mind was occupied with questions I found interesting and relevant; I was on my own and coping fairly well. In short, I felt my own voice was emerging apart from the powerful, but not individual, Rockefeller identity.

The gossip magazine's discovery of my family background undermined such progress. It was not my voice the reporters wanted to broadcast. The emergent self was too fragile to withstand such a barrage. I became reconvinced that people would not want to work with me because my background meant too many hassles and carried too many negative implications. I would never be hired solely on the basis of my own qualifications.

One year later, I decided to no longer use Rockefeller as my last name, and instead began to use my middle name, Dulany. It became tremendously important to me to secure a teaching job without using any Rockefeller-related contacts. Since I was too young to have any other connections, it took me several months to find work. This experience confirmed my suspicion that the only reason I had succeeded at anything in life was because of the Rockefeller connection.

Nevertheless, the alternative school finally hired me, first as a teacher, then as a codirector. This example is not as dramatic as the *favela* story, but it illustrates the consequences of wasting energy and of not having a clear sense of one's own voice.

At the alternative school, I was equally committed to making a difference in these kid's lives—compensating for the lack of love, or fair treatment, or consistent limit-setting they had experienced—and to maintaining my own separate identity as Peggy Dulany, no matter what it cost in my ability to be myself with the students. You may notice some inconsistencies in those two goals.

Most of the students were cynical and mistrustful of adults, while at the same time hungry for role models. They revered my codirector, a man in his 40s, who had grown up in circumstances similar to those of many kids: For instance, he had been in trouble with the law and had hated school. The fact that he had gone through these same experiences and survived with his own distinct voice was a source of hope to them. I felt inadequate in this regard: The stories I could tell that would not give away my family background were not ones with which they could identify. In the perspicacious way adolescents detect insincerity, they must have sensed some falsehood that prolonged their mistrust of me.

Because I really did care about them, consistently set limits, and hung in there for 6 years, I ultimately overcame much of that mistrust. Had I been able to be more honest with them, I might have been more effective.

Of course, if I had approached them as a Rockefeller I would have confronted difficulties of another sort. Poverty was a constant factor in most of their lives, and the emotional deprivation they had suffered often compounded and became confused with the economic deprivation. It would have been hard for them, at least initially, to relate to me with feelings other than hostility and envy. Furthermore, they were so accustomed to blaming all of their problems on lack of money that it would have made them feel very upset and angry to have to face the fact—in the form of my imperfect self—that money does not solve all problems. Nevertheless, if we had overcome that hurdle, I might have been a more complete role model.

In retrospect, I realized that considerable energy was wasted in trying to hide part of myself. The job was draining enough without my adding to its complexity.

After moving from Boston to New York, I began to work at a different job at the New York City Partnership, a private-sector organization whose mission is to make New York City a better place in which to live, work, and do business. The 120 board members are all chief executive officers of organizations that range from large corporations to small businesses, nonprofit groups, and universities.

David Rockefeller chairs the New York City Partnership. I could not possibly work there and hide the fact that I am his daughter. Not only are board members and staff colleagues aware of my family background, but so are the individuals in government, labor, and the community with whom I interact on a daily basis.

I accepted the job at the Partnership just when I had gained a clearer sense of myself; this was no coincidence. Being able to accept the job meant that I was confident that my own voice was strong and clear enough to resonate with its own pitch apart from, yet in concert with, the voices of my father and other co-workers.

Undoubtedly, the variety and quality of my previous experiences contributed to my readiness for this test. Coping, no matter how precariously, with life on my own in Brazil, getting a job on my own at the alternative school, and working through some difficult times gave me concrete evidence of some competence. These varied experiences also provided me opportunities to discover what I like to do, what I did poorly, and what I did well.

ROLE MODELS AND MENTORS

A number of role models along the way, whose voices ring with authenticity, have been critical to the emergence of my own voice. Presenting ideas or arguing philosophy with people whose voices are clear can be intimidating, because it points up so sharply the inconsistencies in one's own thinking. Yet when points are made out of conviction and not for self-aggrandizement, in an effort to reach further clarity rather than to prove one wrong, such role models offer just the kind of challenge and support that hones one's thinking and strengthens one's voice. These mentors coached, cajoled, criticized, and sang along with me until I achieved enough of my own sense of rhythm and tune and lyrics to keep speaking, singing, or shouting on my own, even when the accompaniment stopped.

CONFLICT RESOLUTION

Finding a voice and daring to use it are important first steps. But how do we integrate our belief system with our skills and our professional preferences? The convergence of these factors determines not only our mission in life but how we carry it out.

My mission has changed only slightly over 20 years, but my perception of how I can best carry it out has changed quite dramatically as my voice becomes clearer. My mission is basically to help others find their voices. More specifically, I want to use my understanding of and access to the power structure to broaden it, and to help others who have been disenfranchised gain access through understanding the structure.

In 1987, I founded the Synergos* Institute as yet another step toward this mission. Oriented to solving poverty issues through social action partnerships that bring all those with a stake in the problem to the table, it constitutes yet another way of helping people find their own voice. For who ordinarily does not get heard with regard to their needs? The poor, the disenfranchised—the voiceless. By connecting up my access with an effective institution, we try to ensure that those who normally have no seat at the table have a chair as big as all the others; that those whose voices are normally not heard have a chance to sing as loudly and sweetly as anyone.

Previously, I was unwilling to use my access to empower others. Because I was uncertain about my own personal value, I denied, at least in my professional life, my family's close association with the power structure.

My antipathy toward the discrepancy between the wealthy and the poor also led me to deny my own access and what that could represent in terms of helping others. It was not until I gained more confidence in myself that I was able to recognize that my refusal to take advantage of the privilege into which I was born would not change the way our society operates. However, I realized that I could accomplish more by using my connections to affect our social system so that more people could become empowered. While this particular conflict is perhaps not shared by many, the clarity of voice and effectiveness of action that result from the resolution of internal conflicts are common to all.

After I integrated the different elements of my life into my voice and mission, I still had to come to terms with the discrepancy between what

*Synergos means "working together" in Greek.

I would like to do and what I think I might be able to do. I would like to change the world so that a power structure would be unnecessary, so that there is a truly equal system where all people participate in decisions, regardless of their economic status. After I saw the movie *Gandhi*, it became devastatingly clear that despite an individual's dedication, brilliance, and willingness to sacrifice in the pursuit of a humane and democratic cause, there will always be counterforces that prevent such change.

Extreme fluctuations accompany coming to terms with oneself, particularly in youth. Some years ago, I hoped to have an effect—perhaps a 20% influence—on the 500 high school students whose lives I touched. Even then I experienced some failure. Gradually, we find a comfortable place between extremes, although that place may always be fraught with tensions between competing desires, such as the wish to accomplish the goals of one's larger mission versus the desire to honor more personal commitments. If we use our true voices, these tensions will be minimized by the satisfaction in simultaneously being able to be one's real self and use one's skills to pursue a goal that is personally gratifying and spiritually uplifting.

It is often theorized, however, that women do not form a strong sense of identity in relation to the world until they have settled issues of relationship. While men may derive their identities from their jobs, women have traditionally derived their identities from whom they loved. Whether or not that is good, or even true, we ought to be aware of the implications of following such a pattern.

The voices of men and women have different pitches; if we limit our explorations to the range that overlaps with that of our men, we will probably never discover the sweet pitch that is our own. If we come to a relationship with a voice that is already clear and true, however, it will be much easier to determine with whom we sing the best harmony.

There is a question of balance to be considered here. Certainly one way I define myself is in terms of my relationships. Those bonds—with my son, my friends, my family, my husband—give me courage and strength to pursue my larger mission. Yet if I spend too much time nurturing these relationships, there is no time left for work. If I divide myself entirely between work and relationships, I lose something of the voice that is exclusively mine. I have to add a third category, which is time for myself. During this private time, I rest my voice, consolidate my thinking and feelings, assess how I am doing, and plan what I want to do next. Without that time, I tend to speak without knowing what I want to say, or lean too heavily on my friends, or let my job draw my voice out of me until it no longer resonates with the clarity I am working to achieve. This private time is the key to my ability of maintaining balance and empowerment in that it allows me to further define my voice and establish how I can express it optimally through all components of my life.

ACKNOWLEDGMENT. This chapter is a compendium of segments of two addresses: the Founder's Day address, Spelman College, April 1984, and a commencement speech, Cambridge College, August 1984.

Chapter 10

Mothers Who Abuse Their Children

Virginia N. Wilking

The thought of a woman abusing a child is a terrible one. It contradicts conventional concepts of woman as mother, providing for and protecting her young. Primitive religions, however, recognized a dual role for women by coupling the image of the Great Mother with that of the Destroyer. In these religions goddesses were worshipped cautiously, surrounded by great mystery and reverence, because of their powers over life and death.

In time the furies were given names, transformed into literary characters, and made almost respectable. Woman's aggressive behavior was denied except as an occasional subject of the arts, such as Judith, Medea, Lady MacBeth, or Lucretia Borgia. The concept of the terrible mother was superseded by the gentler concept of the loving mother. The powerful shrieking maenads of Dionysus lost their ascendancy, as virgins and young maidens became socially preferable (Grant, 1962). No longer characterized as avengers or furies, women were portrayed as victims: first held hostage by dragons, later imprisoned in modern doll houses. Although the maenads offer an extreme example, female violence, even child abuse, should not come as a surprise. Current thinking about women recognizes the necessary role that aggression plays in development, and theorists are beginning to trace the origins of destructive rage and aggressive behavior that have escaped the civilizing effect of the developmental process (Nadelson, Notman, Miller, & Zilbach, 1982; Notman, 1982).

VIRGINIA N. WILKING • Columbia University College of Physicians and Surgeons, New York, New York 10032.

WOMEN AND MOTHERS: THE PROBLEM OF THE UNKNOWN

The literature refers to women as parents, as mothers, and as caretakers; one category is frequently substituted for another in thought as well as in the recording of statistics. The prevalence of child abuse in any one of these groups of women is not known. Some women abuse children who are not their own; under these circumstances, the women are caretakers in the bleakest sense of the word. Children may call both biological mothers and caretakers "Mother," combining them in fantasy as "the good mother" and the "bad mother," while separating out the other elements of each woman's life (for example, drugs, a second family, or a job). Women with a predisposing history become child abusers for the same reasons for which they were abused, or they abuse as the result of a multifactorial "circumstance" or overdetermined dynamics. The poor black women I treated in an inner-city municipal hospital abused children in all sorts of ways and for all sorts of reasons. As yet we do not know which women, which children, and which reasons prevail. Investigators have begun to reassess the results of published reports as well as to conduct new studies in an effort to establish a profile of a woman who abuses, although the profile changes with the population studied. Newberger, Newberger, and Hampton (1983) urge that we carefully consider the theoretical construction of knowledge about child abuse as well as the possibility of major methodologic flaws that could limit the usefulness of past and present studies that focus on the abused and the abusers.

PREVALENCE OF ABUSE

The actual prevalence of the abuse of children remains unknown. Schmitt and Kempe (1979) suggest an annual rate of 500 cases in 1 million; this figure includes physical and sexual abuse and failure to thrive. In 1982 the National Center on Child Abuse and Neglect reported that there were 832,000 known cases of child abuse per year; this figure includes 207,000 cases of physical assault, 134,000 cases of emotional abuse, 108,000 cases of physical neglect, and 44,700 cases of sexual abuse. Although in 1983 nearly 1 million cases of child abuse were expected to be reported, the incidence was obviously higher because of underreporting. For example, Gelles (1978) interviewed 2,143 couples who had at least one child between 3 and 17 years of age. Sixty-three percent of the couples reported at least one episode of assault against a child or adolescent during the study year.

In addition to underreporting, another problem lies in the criteria used to identify abuse and to determine who should be responsible for reporting such abuse; the criteria may vary considerably from state to state. Even within the same state, the words *proven, verified,* or *probably* may be defined differently by institutions and agencies. There is a tendency to complicate matters comparable to that found in Dickens's Office of Circumlocution (1894). The staff of one agency refused to accept information about an abused child for whom they were responsible on the basis that the child was dead. In this chapter, I define child abuse as physical and/or sexual abuse inflicted by an adult caretaker on children (up to 11 years old) or adolescents (up to 17 years old).

THE ABUSING WOMAN

The woman who abuses children is more familiar in theory than in fact; the implications of mistreating a child or identifying with the child as "the bad self" (Galdston, 1965), the mother's misperception of the child at the actual moment of abuse (Bishop, 1978), the mother's inability to handle chronic rage and channel even normal aggressive drives into acceptable work, and the mother's perception of the child as monstrous because she feels she has been deprived of contentment (Galdston, 1981) are theoretically acceptable and easily applicable. Indeed, such theories seem to give us more insight into individuals and their feelings than do the facts. Currently, we have only fragmented statistics on the number of women who abuse children. Gil (1968) has reported that, of a sample of 6,000 children, 68% had been abused by their mothers; he suggested this was a function of the greater amount of time that mothers spent with their children. Vesterdal (1979) has reported that 1% of the children in a Swedish study were abused by their mothers and 40% were abused by their fathers. Blumberg (1980) has reported that 70% of the abusers were mothers, while Kinard and Klerman (1980) have reported that women represented 51.8% of the perpetrators in data from the American Humane Society.

Noting that "violence reverberates in the family system," Pascoe and associates (Pascoe, Hebbert, Pearl, & Loda, 1981) have reported that wives were abused in 40 of 132 biological families in which the children were abused. Carmen (1982) has found an incidence of child abuse in at least 20 of 60 families in which wives had been abused. It is not clear if these data will aid our identification of women who abuse children, although it may help in intervention and prevention of child abuse.

ABUSING MOTHERS AND STRESS

Stress has become an increasingly larger umbrella for the specific factors involved in the etiology of child abuse. Green, Gaines, and Sandgrund (1974) have discussed the current environmental stress to which abusing parents are subjected but define these external stresses in terms of the loss of key relationships that surely have their internal representation. Stress widens the gap between the limited capacity of the parent and increased childrearing pressures. According to Green et al., stress is a necessary component in the etiology of child abuse; the other two components are the personality of the parents and the child's own characteristics.

In reviewing the concepts of child abuse between 1972 and 1982, Friedrich and Wheeler (1982) have emphasized the importance of specific stresses and specific biologically determined or learned responses. Their review reflects the growing interest in the nature of the mother–infant interaction. A woman's early social and emotional learning and that of her mother are as important as a woman's biological characteristics. Nature and nurture demand analysis, but, as noted by Newberger et al. (1983) and Gaines, Sangrund, Green, and Power (1978), our methodology, when matched to the complexity of the problem, becomes too complicated and analysis breaks down. The identification of stresses and differentiated and undifferentiated responses poses a problem for researchers.

Abusing mothers often describe stress that they feel drives them to violence. Stress is related to machines and appliances and their breakdown, to people and their hostility, and often to the abused child (Passman & Mulhern, 1977). Specific events may also prove stressful. Altemeier, O'Conner, Vietze, and Sandler (1982) have listed such examples as moving to a new home, the birth of another baby, abuse or desertion by a father, or resigning from a job. Since these are all common to the lives of most women, the specific response that triggers child abuse remains unclear.

Further consideration should be given to certain factors that strongly influence abusing mothers: poverty, single parenthood, and age. All three of these factors involve external and internal stress.

POVERTY AND ABUSING MOTHERS

Although not all studies prove the relationship between poverty and child abuse, more child abuse is reported among poor families. Pelton (1978) has noted a greater incidence of abuse, as well as the worst degree of abuse, including the highest mortality rate, among the poorest classes. Pelton's paper on the myth of classlessness in child abuse followed an interest in the fact that child abuse was not limited to the poor, a view that obscures the misery of poverty and the specific stresses to which it gives rise. Among the poor, the mothers usually assume the responsibility of trying to buy food and clothing for the family with too little money. Thus, the external circumstance of poverty engenders feelings of low self-esteem, anger, and resentment, and the dependent child creates the circumstance in which needs and demands act as specific stressors.

Gil (1968) has reported on child abuse in all socioeconomic classes but has noted a greater incidence in poor urban areas. Observing that most of the families they studied lived comfortably, Silver, Dublin, and Lourie (1969) consider a history of child abuse to be stronger predictor than that of family income. Although Spinetta (1978) has argued that certain personality traits and attitudes may predispose individuals of any social class to violence, he did not consider it contradictory that the greatest incidence of child abuse has been reported among the lowest class. Altemeier et al. (1982) have found no evidence that supported the relationship between social class and abuse in a follow-up of a prenatal clinic population. Nevertheless, Shearman, Evans, Boyle, Cuddy, and Norman (1983) and Elmer (1977) have found poverty to be a contributing factor, and Murphy, Jenkins, Newcomb, and Sibert (1981) have used it as a criterion for prediction and intervention. Thus, while the abusing mother can come from any social class, in 50 to 80% of the cases of abused reported she is poor (Pelton, 1978).

The Abusing Mother as a Single Parent

Before the dramatic increase in single-parent families, mothers living alone with their children, usually in lower-class families, were considered to be at high risk for becoming abusers. Although today a mother alone seems less remarkable, the nature of the single-parent home warrants analysis. This analysis should take into consideration the man who may live in the home or the transient father.

In early and mid-adolescence, single parenthood is not a natural state, but being single is a normal circumstance. The late adolescents appear to face the greatest risk because they may be in charge of their own households, even if the children spend most of the day with grandparents. Thus, the stresses of single parenthood as well as the usual stresses of adolescence come into play.

Ounsted, Gordon, and Milligan (1982) have reported that 37% of 7,108 mothers who were referred from an obstetrical service because they were considered to be at risk for becoming child abusers were single parents. (Ounsted did not correlate single parenthood with income level.)

AGE AND STAGE OF DEVELOPMENT

The age of an abusing mother may not reflect her developmental stage. A 13-year-old girl, acting out sexually, does not suddenly become a young woman when she has a baby at 14 years, and she should not be described as such. The demands made on her by society and her family are sources of stress, because they are at odds with her developmental tasks. The unconscious longings expressed through pregnancy are not limited to early adolescents, but the disappointment of these girls often is particularly acute. The 14-year-old really thought she could become the baby, the 13-year-old really wanted something to love, the 15-year-old thought she could replace her brother killed in Vietnam. Thus, babies frequently become the natural victims of young mothers' rage, disappointment, and despair.

Bolton, Laner, and Kane (1980) have reported that younger mothers did not abuse more frequently except in lower socioeconomic classes. Blumberg (1980) regards youth as an important factor in child abuse when related to single-parent status. In analyzing the figures of the American Humane Society, Kinard and Klerman (1980) have found the same figure for abuse among older and younger women and could not substantiate the work of Murphy and associates (1981), who view age as an important predictor for younger mothers at risk. Shearman et al. (1983) have reported that in a group of 86 children and their mothers, there were three times as many abusing mothers as there were control subjects below the age of 18. The findings, however, were not statistically significant, with the mean age of abusing mothers at 22 years and that of the control group at 25.

In a Georgia study of 2,281 abused children and their parents (Child Abuse in Georgia, 1979), the mean age of the abuser was reported at 30 years, for both fathers and mothers. Lynch and Roberts (1977) have reported that the age of the mother at the time of the birth of her first child is more important than her age at the time the abuse of a child occurred.

NATURE, TRAITS, AND ATTITUDES

The nature of abusing mothers has been under observation since the first reports on child abuse appeared in the literature in the early 1960s. With careful analysis of the interaction between mother and child, we may be ending where Morris and Gould (1963) began. Wasserman, Green, and Allen (1983) noted that abusing parents turned to their children, reversing the pattern of emotional dependency. Steele and

Pollack (1968) emphasized the mother's unreal expectations and unsuccessful relationships. Kempe and Helfer (1972) pointed out that a mother's early lack of nurturance could limit her ability to love.

Initially, researchers attempted to explain the aberrations of the abusing mother in terms of herself. The view of the mother as a loving woman lingered but was poorly defined; by specifying personality traits, first in provocative small studies and then in larger definitive studies, we will learn more about the nature of abusing mothers, and thus be able to help mothers prevent abuse. The study of these attributes does not rule out the importance of thinking in multifactorial terms; rather, it should improve our study of the interaction of maternal or parental character, the child's character, and stress. While investigators have focused on self-esteem, overidentification of mother and child, poor emotional control and anger, and the nature of maternal expectations, they have not yet fully explored the effects of depression, so common among lower-class mothers who abuse.

SELF-ESTEEM

Rosen and Stein (1980) emphasize the absence of self-esteem in abusing mothers. The relationship between self-esteem and the sublimation of aggression into successful mothers (Notman, 1982) has also been underscored. Sharkey (1980) has found that self-esteem was rated higher than expected in the population studies. Kaplan, Pelcovitz, and Salzinger (1983) suggest that this finding represents the abusing mother's conscious choice of a more socially acceptable answer on which she is to be commended.

OVERIDENTIFICATION

An abusing mother's overidentification with her child and the implication of her confusion about self and nonself are difficult to explore. A statistical, controlled approach to the unconscious is not beyond us but is extremely complicated. Attempts to destroy the bad self are familiar to us from the dynamics of suicidal patients with only slight modifications; such attempts to search and destroy can be applied to the dynamics of child abuse. Twentyman and Plotkin (1982) discuss the psychopathological projections of abusing mothers, including their suspicions of others. IF investigators trace the relationship of the abusing mother and child back to early childhood, they may uncover evidence of a pathological turning point when normal symbiosis and closeness became abnormal.

Abusing Mothers and Controls

The problem of impulse control among abusing mothers is multi-faceted. Some investigators focus on the mother only and some on the mother in relation to the abused child. Blumberg (1980) and Herrenkohl and Herrenkohl (1979) agree that an abusing mother's control over impulse and violence is poor. Spinetta and Rigler (1972) describe abusing mothers as impulse-ridden while emphasizing their wish to be in control (Spinetta, 1978); Rosen and Stein (1980) underline the value they give to authority, and Galdston (1981) sees abusing mothers as menaced by their child, which is out of their control. Abusing mothers have been described as angry and lonely (Spinetta, 1978). Green, Liang, Gaines, and Sultan (1980) have noted their disorganized anger. The contribution of Wasserman et al. (1983) is probably the most helpful in reporting on the nuances of control and compliance in 12 abusing mother–infant pairs. They observed that abusing mothers' behavior did not differ from that of nonabusing mothers except in an increased tendency toward physical contact; such studies should be replicated to keep investigators honest in their approaches.

Abusing Mother's Expectations

The abusing mother's expectations of her children during the course of childrearing have also been approached from several points of view. Passman and Mulhern (1977), Twentyman and associates (1982), and Vesterdal (1979) agree that the expectations of abusing mothers are unrealistic. Twentyman et al. (1982) indicate that educational deficits explain the lack of realism. Spinetta (1978) writes of the qualitative differences in the expectations. A child might meet the mother's expectations under certain circumstances, but Rosen and Stein (1980) have pointed out that such expectations may vacillate with a mother's inconsistencies. In reviewing the work of Spinetta and Rigler (1972) 10 years later, Friedrich and Wheeler (1982) suggest that abusing mothers do not lack knowledge of childrearing practices but lack knowledge of their child.

This area of predictive traits and attributes is a disheartening one. Although a characteristic, possibly related statistically to the occurrence of abuse in a specific group of mothers, has been painstakingly teased out of its psychological matrix, the studies do not weave all of the psychological threads together again.

Despite the considerable number of mothers who abuse their children, relatively few have a formal psychiatric diagnosis and relatively few are seen for full evaluation. While Vesterdal (1979) refers to "psychological disturbance" as a factor in abuse in Sweden, Lynch and Roberts (1977) use emotional disturbances as a criterion in identifying mothers at risk; Ounsted et al. (1982) use psychiatric history under similar circumstances.

In a recent study, Kaplan et al. (1983) evaluated 76 abusing mothers and have reported finding considerably more psychopathology, including depressive disorders, alcoholism, drug abuse, antisocial personality, and labile personality, among the abusing mothers than among the 38 nonabusing control subjects. None of the abusing mothers was given a diagnosis of schizophrenia. In reporting on a group of abusing parents, Galdston (1965) has used the term *transient psychosis* to emphasize the gap in reality testing and the failures in integregation at the time of abuse. Despite the quantity of papers on child abuse, few have dealt with exact diagnosis. Thus, the profile of the abusing mother remains poorly articulated, although some of the features may be familiar. In drawing such profiles, one must remember Robert Benchley, who, after drawing the features of the archcriminal with a flourish, realized he had sketched a picture of himself.

THE CHILD WHO IS ABUSED

In 1964 Milowe and Lourie wrote that a defect in the child had to be considered as a factor in abuse; for example, the child might be unresponsive or have other personality traits that invite abuse from a specific mother. In 1965 Galdston described the abused child as incapable of improper response. Then interest in the child as a factor in the etiology of child abuse lapsed until the 1970s. Green, Gaines, Sandgrund, and Haberfield (1974), however, have continued to write in detail about the abused child. As with the abusing mother, no one characteristic identified the abused child. Often, the mother's violence, directed toward another person, is, in turn, projected upon the child. For example, the mother may misperceive and see the child as her own abusing mother, or simply misperceive the child's behavior as provocative, punishing, or disobedient.

Infants and young children are dependent on their adult caretakers and thus are extremely vulnerable. An estimated 32% of all child abuse is directed toward infants under 1 year old; 61% of the cases involve children under 3 (Pascoe et al., 1981). Other figures indicate that adolescents between 12 and 17 years of age could account for an estimated 38% of the abuse (Smith & Hanson, 1974), leaving the abused child of middle childhood squeezed between these two sets of somewhat incompatible statistics. The reasons for and the nature of abuse in adolescence depend on whether or not it began in early childhood.

Silver et al. (1969) have suggested that abusing parents abuse children of all ages. The number of young infants abused, however, indicates that the demands made by this age group on the mother create a particular problem.

The sex of the child most frequently abused varies with the report; the numbers of girls and boys abused are probably near equal. Gil (1968) has reported that more than 50% were boys; in contrast, in a study conducted in Georgia (Child Abuse in Georgia, 1979), the Center for Disease Control reports that more girls were abused. The extent of the abuse remains an important variable. It may vary with intent, with accident, with age of the child, and with criteria used to rate severity of abuse; for instance, terms such as *verified* and *confirmed* do not describe the seriousness of abuse the way mortality figures do. Gil (1968) describes 53% of the cases reviewed in his demographic survey as "not serious," yet in 60% of the cases, children were abused repeatedly. Schmitt and Kempe (1979) report that 5% of the children die of subsequent abuse if returned home after legal intervention, and 35% are seriously injured under similar circumstances.

Smith and Hanson (1974) have reported that one-half of the cases in a study of 134 children were seriously abused; 21 died and 35 were battered more than once. Mitchell (1975) has reported 5,000 cases of child abuse per year in the United Kingdom, of whom 5 to 10% die and 25% show residual disability, compared with approximately 2,000 deaths per year in the United States (Schmitt & Kempe, 1979). On the other hand, Martin, Breezley, Conway, and Kempe (1974) do not describe major neurological and other serious residual effects in the follow-up of 58 American children, and Elmer (1977) has found, to her surprise, that a group of abused children evaluated after 17 years were not very different from the control group. Green, Gaines, Sandgrund, and Haberfield (1974) have taken a more serious view of the damage done in terms of mental retardation and psychological damage and have described the coping mechanism of abused children as maladaptive (Green, 1983).

Although children may physically survive abuse, their psychological survival is questionable. The "frozen watchfulness" (Ounsted, Oppenheimer, & Lindsay, 1974) and the "unnaturalness" (Elmer, 1960) of abused children bode ill for their future and cast the same shadow on the next generation that has been cast on the present one.

The effects of abuse on a child's development requires further study. Herrenkohl and Herrenkohl (1979) have compared abused children with their siblings and have discovered no differences between them. Friedrich and Boriskin (1976) note they may be "different" but are primarily considered different by their mothers, to whom they have special meaning as part of a complex interaction. Green, Liang, Gaines, and Sultan (1980) include this special meaning in their examples of children's characteristics that were part of the etiology of abuse. Biological, characterological, and developmental defects, such as mental retardation or speech impediments, have been stressed and viewed with proper alarm but remain only factors. External stresses for development include those that crowd or pressure the abusing mothers: poverty, malnutrition, or frequent illness, for example. More important are the implications of nature rather than nurture in early infancy—that is, of the infant's innate temperament (Blumberg, 1980) or failure to understand signals that raise the question of a defect in the child, as Milowe and Lourie (1964) have theorized.

Problems in Bonding

Ounsted et al. (1974) attributed the mothers' earlier parenting failures to failures in symbiosis mentioned by Vesterdal (1979). In contrast, Coppolillo (1979) has emphasized the mother's sense of isolation and her failure to feel the reward of motherliness. Roberts, Lynch, and Golding (1980) have noted that abusing mothers are "not engrossed"; similarly, Wasserman et al. (1983) have found a lack of mutual pleasure among abusing mothers and their children. As noted earlier, Galdston (1981) describes abusing mothers as having deprived themselves of the experience of contentment. Thus, their abused children adjust to a sadomasochistic relationship.

Intervention and Research Needs

After observing mothers and their infants, Wasserman et al. (1983) have documented disordered interaction and suggested research methodology. They discuss possible interventions that involved changing a baby's responses, which, in turn, would serve as a catalyst to change the mother's responses. Egeland and Sroufe (1981) indicated that in the treatment of nonabusing but at-risk mother–infant pairs, it is possible to alter the infant's attachment relationship and thus improve its resilience and resistance to change.

Researchers should pursue the following goals to build a more comprehensive data base on child abuse: Improvement in the recording and correlation of comparable data from each state, use of information available through the psychoanalytic treatment of small numbers of patients, standardization of the interactions of mother–infant pairs, and continuation of studies of disturbed interaction between abusing mother and child are essential. Further definition of the actions of abusing parents is equally important. Controlled prospective studies, at-risk population studies, and follow-up of abused children that will record their behavior as parents should be carried out.

Intervention between parents and their abused children began with the first formal reports, characterized by the difficulty the abusing mothers have in trusting, in lowering family resistance against interference, and in initiating and maintaining relationships. Individual psychiatric treatment, counseling, peer groups, and support from families and community workers have been used to help abusing parents; all of these interventions are slow and time-consuming. With studies such as those by Green et al. (1980) it has become clear that abused children need far more help, with their mothers and individually, than they have received. Abused preschool children, for example, require the daily support of a therapeutic nursery in which their mothers participate. Although some investigators report enthusiastic response to various kinds of help, including clinic follow-up visits, supportive interviews, and use of consultants (Altmeier et al., 1982; Ounsted et al., 1974, 1982), others note considerable lack of interest, broken appointments, and failure to accept help.

At the far end of the scale of interventions for abused children lies placement outside of the home. A mother who is afraid of abusing her child further may opt for voluntary placement, but these arrangements often prove unrealistic. Frequently the child asks to return home prematurely. Involuntary placement is carried out only for the 20% of abused children seen by the court; of these, 5 to 10% are placed in what Runyan, Gould, Trost, and Loda (1981) consider to be an extremely haphazard fashion.

Prediction of abuse and identification of at-risk mothers, usually with young infants, have been suggested as a national public health campaign in England and the United States. Murphy et al. (1981), Shearman et al. (1983), and Altemeier et al. (1982) have initiated such projects, using simple criteria, such as the mother's age and social class, her history of emotional disturbance, and the admission of the infant to a special unit (Murphy et al., 1981).

Despite these efforts, much remains to be done. How could we have helped Ms. V, who broke her 7-year-old daughter's arm in a second episode of abuse? Three years after this incident, Ms. V wanted her daughter returned to her by the court. Ms. V said she was sure she would not abuse her daughter again; she said she would be a fool to do so, and anyway her daughter was older.

Smartly dressed in a red jumpsuit, Ms. V showed little concern about her daughter but was interested in her formal return. In fact, the daughter had been living unofficially with Ms. V during most of the 3-year separation, instead of with her maternal grandmother. When asked why she had not had another child, Ms. V said, "If I have a second child, I might not have had enough money to dress her and might feel bad, looking at my own nice clothes."

Abused children like Ms. V's daughter must be helped in time for the next generation. These children will remember their parenting, having suffered from the nature of their parent's parenting, and without proper intervention will carry their childhood of abuse into their adult lives, becoming abusers themselves. The needs and afflictions of mothers like Ms. V must also be addressed for the betterment of their own welfare and that of their children.

REFERENCES

Altemeier, W. A., O'Conner, S., Vietze, P. M., & Sandler, H. M. (1982). Antecedents of a child abuse. *Journal of Pediatrics, 100,* 823–829.

Bishop, F. J. (1978). The abusing parents: Perceptions, memories and pathological identification as precipitants in the attack. In E. J. Anthony, C. Koupernik, & C. Chiland (Eds.), *The child in his family: Vulnerable children.* New York: Wiley.

Blumberg, M. L. (1980). The abusing mother: Criminal, psychopath or victim of circumstances. *American Journal of Psychotherapy, 34,* 351–362.

Bolton, F. J., Jr., Laner, R. H., & Kane, S. P. (1980). Child maltreatment risk among adolescent mothers. A study of reported cases. *American Journal of Orthopsychiatry, 50,* 489–504.

Carmen, E. (1982). Wife abuse: Culture as destiny. In M. T. Notman & C. C. Nadelson (Eds.), *Development and Stresses, Vol. 3.* New York: Plenum Press.

Child abuse in Georgia 1975–1977. (1979). *Journal of the Medical Association of Georgia, 68,* 393–394.

Coppolillo, H. (1978). A conceptual model for study of some abusing parents. In E. J. Anthony, C. Koupernik, and C. Chiland (Eds.), *Vulnerability and parenthood. The child and his family* Vol. 4, (pp. 231–238). New York: Wiley.

Dickens, C. (1894). *Little Dorrit* (p. 111). Boston and New York: Houghton Mifflin.

Egeland, B., & Sroufe, L. A. (1981). Attachment and early maltreatment. *Child Development, 52,* 44–52.

Elmer, E. A. (1960). Abused young children seen in hospitals. *Social Work, 5,* 98–100.

Elmer, E. A. (1977). Follow-up study of traumatized children. *Pediatrics, 59,* 273–279.

Friedrich, W. N., & Boriskin, J. A. (1976). The role of the child in abuse: A review of the literature. *American Journal of Orthopsychiatry, 46,* 580–590.

Friedrich, W. M., & Wheeler, K. K. (1982). The abusing parent revisited: A decade of psychological research. *Journal of Nervous and Mental Disease, 170,* 577–587.

Gaines, R., Sandgrund, A., Green, A. H., & Power, E. (1978). Etiological factors in child maltreatment: A multivariate study of abusing, neglecting and normal mothers. *Journal of Abnormal Psychology, 87*(5), 531–540.

Galdston, R. (1965). Observations on children who have been physically abused and their parents. *American Journal of Psychiatry, 122,* 440–443.

Galdston, R. (1981). The domestic dimensions of violence: Child abuse. *Psychoanalytic Study of the Child, 36,* 391–414.

Gelles, R. J. (1978). Violence toward children. *American Journal of Orthopsychiatry, 48,* 580–592.

Gil, D. (1968). Incidence of child abuse and demographic characteristics of persons involved. In R. Helfer & C. Kempe (Eds.), *The battered child*. Chicago: University of Chicago Press.

Grant, M. C. (1962). *Myths of the Greeks and Romans* (p. 278). Cleveland and New York: World.

Green, A. H. (1983). Child abuse: Dimensions of psychological trauma in abused children. *Journal of the American Academy of Child Psychiatry, 22*, 231–237.

Green, A. H., Gaines, R. W., & Sandgrund, A. (1974). Child abuse: Pathological syndrome of family interaction. *American Journal of Psychiatry, 131*, 882–886.

Green, A. H., Gaines, R. W., Sandgrund, A., & Haberfield, H. (1974, May). *Psychological sequelae of child abuse and neglect*. Paper presented at the meeting of the American Psychiatric Association, Detroit.

Green, A. H., Liang, V., Gaines, R., & Sultan, S. (1980). Psychopathological assessment of child abusing. Neglecting and normal mothers. *Journal of Nervous and Mental Disease, 168*, 356–360.

Herrenkohl, E. C., & Herrenkohl, R. C. (1979). A comparison of abused children and their non-abused siblings. *Journal of the American Academy of Child Psychiatry, 18*, 260–269.

Kaplan, S. J., Pelcovitz, D., & Salzinger, S. (1983). Psychopathology of parents of abused and neglected children and adolescents. *Journal of the American Academy of Child Psychiatry, 22*, 238–244.

Kempe, C., & Helfer, R. E. (Eds.). (1972). *Helping the battered child and his family*. Philadelphia: Lippincott.

Kinard, E. M., & Klerman, L. V. (1980). Teenage parenting and child abuse: Are they related. *American Journal of Orthopsychiatry, 50*, 481–488.

Lynch, M. A., & Roberts, J. (1977). Predicting child abuse: Signs of bonding failure in the maternity hospital. *British Medical Journal, 1*(6061), 624–626.

Martin, H. P., Beezley, P., Conway, E. F., & Kempe, C. H. (1974). The development of abused children: A review of the literature and physical, neurologic, and intellectual findings. *Advances in Pediatrics, 21*, 25–73.

Milowe, I. D., & Lourie, R. S. (1964). The child's role in the battered child syndrome. *Journal of Pediatrics, 65*, 1075–1081.

Mitchell, R. G. (1975). The incidence and nature of child abuse. *Developmental Medicine and Child Neurology, 17*(5), 641–646.

Morris, M., & Gould, R. (1963). A necessary concept in dealing with the "battered child syndrome." *American Journal of Orthopsychiatry, 33*, 298–299.

Murphy, I. F., Jenkins, J., Newcomb, R. G., & Sibert, J. R. (1981). Objective birth data and the prediction of child abuse. *Archives of Disease in Childhood, 56*, 295–297.

Nadelson, C. C., Notman, M. T., Miller, J. B., & Zilbach, J. (1982). Aggression in women: Conceptual issues and clinical implications. In M. T. Notman & C. C. Nadelson (Eds.), *Aggression, adaptations, and psychotherapy*. New York: Plenum Press.

Newberger, E. G., Newberger, C. M., & Hampton, R. H. (1983). Child abuse: The current theory base and future research needs. *Journal of the American Academy of Child Psychiatry, 22*, 262–268.

Notman, M. T. (1982). Feminine development: Changes in psychoanalytic theory. In M. T. Notman & C. C. Nadelson (Eds.), *Concepts of femininity and the life cycle*. New York: Plenum Press.

Ory, M. G., & Earp, J. A. (1981). Child maltreatment and the use of social services. *Public Health Report, 96*, 238–245.

Ounsted, C., Gordon, J. C., & Milligan, B. (1982). Fourth goal of perinatal medicine. *British Medical Journal, 284*, 879–885.

Ounsted, C., Oppenheimer, R., & Lindsay, J. (1974). Aspects of bonding failure: The psychological and psychotherapeutic treatment of families of battered children. *Developmental Medicine and Child Neurology, 16*, 447–456.

Pascoe, J. M., Hebbert, V., Pearl, T. M., & Loda, F. (1981). Violence in North Carolina families referred to a child protection team. *North Carolina Medical Journal, 42*, 35–37.

Passman, R. H., & Mulhern, R. K. (1977). Maternal punitiveness as affected by situational stress. An experimental analogue of child abuse. *Journal of Abnormal Psychology, 86*, 565–569.

Pelton, L. (1978). Child abuse and neglect: The myth of classlessness. *American Journal of Orthopsychiatry, 48*, 608–617.

Roberts, J., Lynch, M. A., & Golding, J. (1980). Postneonatal mortality in children from abusing families. *British Journal of Medicine, 281*(6233), 102–104.

Rosen, B., & Stein, M. T. (1980). Women who abuse their children: Implications for pediatric practice. *American Journal of Diseases of Children, 134*, 947–950.

Runyan, D. K., Gould, C. L., Trost, D. L., & Loda, F. A. (1981). Determinants of foster care placement for the maltreated child. *American Journal of Public Health, 71*, 706–711.

Schmitt, B. D., & Kempe, C. H. (1979). Neglect and abuse of children. In V. C. Vaughn, R. J. Mckay, & R. E. Behrman (Eds.), *Nelson's textbook of pediatrics* (11th ed., p. 120). Philadelphia: W. B. Saunders.

Sharkey, C. T. (1980). Sense of personal worth, self-esteem and anomia of child abusing mothers and control. *Journal of Clinical Psychology, 36*, 817–820.

Shearman, J. K., Evans, C. E., Boyle, M. H., Cuddy, L. J., & Norman, G. R. (1983). Maternal and infant characteristics in abuse: A case control study. *Journal of Family Practice, 16*, 289–293.

Silver, L. B., Dublin, C. G., & Lourie, R. S. (1969). Does violence breed violence. Contributions from a study of the child abuse syndrome. *American Journal of Psychiatry, 126*, 404–407.

Smith, S. M., & Hanson, R. (1974). 134 battered children: A medial and psychological study. *British Medical Journal, 3*, 666–670.

Spinetta, J. J. (1978). Parental personality factors in child abuse. *Journal of Consulting and Clinical Psychology, 46*, 1409–1414.

Spinetta, J. J., & Rigler, D. (1972). The child abusing parent: A psychological review. *Psychological Bulletin, 77*, 296–304.

Steele, B. F., & Pollack, C. (1968). A psychiatric study of parents who abuse infants and small children. In R. E. Helfer & C. H. Kempe (Eds.), *The battered child*. Chicago: University of Chicago Press.

Twentyman, C. T., & Plotkin, R. C. (1982). Unrealistic expectations. *Journal of Clinical Psychology, 38*, 497–503.

Vesterdal, J. (1979). Psychological mechanisms in child-abusing parents. *Pediatrician, 8*, 145–151.

Wasserman, G. A., Green, A., & Allen, R. (1983). Good beyond abuse: Maladaptive patterns of interaction in abusing mother–infant pairs. *Journal of the American Academy of Child Psychiatry, 22*, 245–252.

Chapter 11

Female Offenders

ELISSA P. BENEDEK

The female offender has existed since Medea. She has been considered by those interested in crime and criminals as an aberration, a minority. Recently, in the media, academics (sociologists, psychiatrists, and psychologists) and lay authors have emphasized dramatic increases in the prevalence and incidence of female crime. They also have commented on an increasing variety in the spectrum of offenses committed by women. Statistical data that support an increase in female crime are controversial. The theory that a massive increase in female crime comes as a result of women's liberation also is controversial. It is clear and noncontroversial that as large numbers of women are being apprehended, sentenced, placed on probation, or incarcerated, the programs available to female offenders have changed very little. Programming does not meet their needs.

This chapter comments first on the extent of female criminality, then considers existing theoretical perspectives on crime and delinquency from a psychological, biological, and sociological viewpoint. After addressing the spectrum of crimes committed by girls and women, the chapter focuses on females in the correctional system and prisons.

STATISTICS

The actual extent of female crime and delinquency continues to be difficult to determine. The best available data on female crime come from the *Uniform Crime Reports* produced by the Federal Bureau of Investigation. There are numerous problems associated with this data source. Sutherland and Cressy (1978) discuss in depth six reasons why crime as

---

ELISSA P. BENEDEK • Center for Forensic Psychiatry, Ann Arbor, Michigan 48106.

measured by the FBI and reflected in the *Uniform Crime Reports* measures only a small portion of criminal behavior.

1. For a variety of reasons, many persons do not report crime. This is especially true of crimes committed against women. Crime often is not reported by women victims who have been brutalized and humiliated and are ashamed. In most crimes of violence, the victims are women, the victimizers are men.

2. Police may underarrest criminals in some jurisdictions for political reasons—i.e., to make it appear as if crime is decreasing. Conversely, they may inflate arrest figures or overarrest. A crackdown on crime (for example, a crackdown on prostitution) may lead to a massive increase in arrest figures for this crime, which is often victimless.

3. Some crimes, such as homicide, receive more attention or are more apt to be discovered than others. Thus, statistics for homicide may be accurate, but white-collar crimes are less likely to be discovered or, if discovered, less likely to be handled in the criminal justice system.

4. Improvement in law enforcement mechanisms, increases in the number of personnel, more efficient training of police in crime detection and investigation, highly specialized police divisions, and organized drives against crimes tend to increase the number of potential arrests. During the period when the Law Enforcement Administration Agency was operating at full strength, public funds were invested in improving law enforcement mechanisms. The increase in both technology and person power greatly added to the number of arrests and convictions.

5. The 50 states and the District of Columbia vary in their classification of crime. This affects the number of crimes known to and reported by the police. Indeed, the *Uniform Crime Reports* are not uniform. A crime may be classified as a felony in one location, a misdemeanor in another. It may be called homicide in one jurisdiction and manslaughter in another.

6. Crime and arrest rates are computed on the basis of census and enumerated general population figures that fail to take into account changes in the population every 10 years by a census that consistently underrates ethnic groups, especially Afro-Americans (Sutherland and Cressey, 1978).

Rans (1978) raises many additional questions about the validity and reliability of the *Uniform Crime Reports*. She comments that the number of law enforcement agencies and the estimated total population in the FBI samples vary from year to year and from table to table, making each year's data not *exactly* comparable to past years' data or other tables. She reminds us that the ability of law enforcement agencies to gather, report, and record crime and arrest statistics has improved markedly since 1960. Many early statistics did not record female arrests separately from male arrests. Data on women's arrests in particular often were underreported or inaccurate. With the rapid advancement of computer technology and expansion of recordkeeping personnel, more data have been captured. Finally, arrest tables never have been adjusted for changes in the classification of many property crimes from misdemeanor to felony due to inflation.

It is obvious there are serious difficulties with the best available data we have to depict the crime problem in general. It is equally evident that male participation in crime and delinquency has been documented more clearly.

The FBI *Uniform Crime Reports* is divided into Part I and Part II offenses, depending on the seriousness of the crime committed. The Part I offenses are categorized into violent crime (murder, forcible rape, aggravated assault, and robbery) and property crimes (burglary, larceny, theft, arson, and motor vehicle theft). The less serious or nonindexed Part II offenses are other offenses, such as simple assault, forgery and counterfeiting, fraud, embezzlement, prostitution and commercialized vices, sex offenses, drug abuse violations, offenses against the family and children (including nonsupport, neglect, desertion, and abuse), driving under the use of liquor or narcotics, disorderly conduct, and curfew and loitering, which apply only to juveniles and runaways.

According to FBI uniform crime statistics, in the past 20 years, female arrests as the proportion of total arrests have not varied by more than 5 percentage points. In 1960 females constituted 10.7% of the total number of arrested persons; by 1975 they were 15.7% of that total. Nor has the type of offense for which females are arrested fluctuated over this time span. The female crime of today mirrors the female crime of yesteryear. The increase in the rates of arrests for females resulted mainly from increases in property crimes, especially larceny. The increase in the rates of arrests for females for violent crimes was similar to that for males. In summarizing data on female offenders, the *Report to the Nation on Crime and Justice* (1980) says: "Men commit more crimes and are arrested for more serious crimes. Arrest, jail and prison data all suggest women have a stronger relative involvement than men in property crimes such as larceny, forgery, fraud and embezzlement, and in drug offenses. Men are more likely than women to be involved in robbery or burglary" (p. 35).

In both jail and prison, burglary was the charge or conviction for 19% of the men but only 5% of the women. These proportions were reversed in the cases of forgery, fraud, and embezzlement. Almost twice the proportion of women to men were incarcerated for some type of drug offense.

Unfortunately, there is a popular belief (Adler, 1975; Simon, 1975) that women's criminality is becoming similar to the criminality of men, especially where violent and aggressive crimes are concerned. The media have created a new superstar, the female criminal. (Patty Hearst, Jean Harris, and Squeaky Fromm were media sensations and not reflective of the general pattern of female crime.)

THEORETICAL AND CONCEPTUAL PERSPECTIVES OF FEMALE CRIMINALITY

In an attempt to explain women's involvement in criminal behavior, the theoretical literature focuses mainly on four major topics—biology, psychology, social roles, and socioeconomics. Between 1875 and 1926, 15 studies of cacogenic families were published, including the classic studies of the Jukes and the Kallikak families (Weisheit, 1984). In analyzing these studies, Hahn (1980) concluded that women were portrayed as primary initiators and transmitters of biological flaws directly associated with the criminality of women and their family members. In other words, there was direct genetic transmission of criminal behavior.

At the turn of the century, Lombroso and Ferrero (1916) offered another early biological explanation of female criminality. He constructed a developmental hierarchy of superiority involving racial and sexual variables. The hierarchy ranged from the most highly developed (white males) to the most primitive (nonwhite females). He explained all crime as the result of inborn atavistic traits reflecting primitiveness of development. Lombroso postulated that women and savages shared many traits, and he concluded that all criminal women were deficient in a moral sense. He explained women's lesser involvement in criminal behavior as the result of their lower intelligence; ascribed to deviant criminal females a tendency to be cruel, vengeful, and jealous; identified certain physical stigmata or anomalies that were alleged to be characteristic of the more primitive or apelike species of men and women; and believed that offenders exhibited four or more of such anomalies. For example, a prehensile foot, large jaws, outstanding ears, large cheekbones, long arms, and hairiness were all considered atavistic biological throwbacks in the subhuman type, or so-called born criminals. Lombroso and his son-in-law, W. Ferrero (1916), published a study arguing that biological factors led to unusually sinister forms of criminality in women.

> We have seen that the normal woman is naturally less sensitive to pain than man. We also saw that women have many traits in common with children; that their moral sense is deficient; that they are revengeful, jealous, and inclined to vengeances of a refined cruelty.
>
> In ordinary cases these defects are neutralized by piety, maternity, wanton passion, sexual coldness, weakness and an underdeveloped intelligence. But when a morbid activity of the physical centers intensified the bad qualities of women, and induces them to seek relief in evil deeds . . . it is

clear that the innocuous semi criminal present in the normal woman must be transformed into a born criminal more terrible than any man . . . the criminal woman is consequently a monster. (pp. 150–152)

Lombroso and Ferrero (1916) also examined the skulls and bones of deceased female prisoners for signs of atavism and compared them with controls of normal women. They observed that "fallen women" or criminals had the smallest cranial capacity of all and that the brains of female criminals weighed less than those of normal women. Lombroso and Ferrero also described female criminals as shorter, heavier, precociously gray, with darker hair and eyes, longer hands, bigger calves, and a longer jaw than normal women.

Thomas (1907) also wrote about the importance of the weight of the female brain. He, however, did not connect brain size to intelligence, noting that differences in intellectual functioning not only were biologically based but were influenced by the social milieu. In his book *The Unadjusted Girl* (1923), Thomas broke with Lombroso's biological theories and discussed the influence of the social environment on deviant behavior. In describing a study of 647 prostitutes, he observed that their socioeconomic status, deplorable home conditions, and lack of education might be reasons for their becoming prostitutes.

More recently, Dalton (1980) has studied the role of menstruation and premenstrual tension in violent criminal behavior. Her studies document her belief that violent behavior in women is linked to the premenstrum. She studied a sample of women inmates in an English women's prison and observed that these women committed crimes during either the menstrual period or premenstrum. Her methodology and conclusions have been criticized severely by Benedek (1985), Holtzman (1984), and Horney (1978).

Pollak (1950) served as a bridge between biological theorists and sociological theorists, arguing that criminality of women began with their natural deceitfulness. He alleged that the female anatomy and physiology allowed and encouraged women to practice deceit more readily than males; that is, a man "could not conceal an erection" but a woman could conceal sexual arousal, interest, or lack of interest in sexuality. Pollak suggested that the menstrual cycle and the secrecy surrounding it also was a basic biological difference that led to a woman's natural deceitfulness. He believed that the generative phases of women—"menstruation, pregnancy, and menopause," each of which is dramatically influenced by hormonal changes—are precursors to deviant female behavior. Further, Pollak suggested that chivalry on the part of men in the criminal justice system is responsible for the fact that few women ever were charged by the police for their crimes, and, if charged, such women were either acquitted or given shorter sentences.

Contemporary efforts to explain female criminal behavior have focused more on gender role, social role, and socioeconomic factors. Adler (1975) argued that women were emancipated in the United States and the Western world, and because of their emancipation they were entering into new masculine areas of experience. Their new freedom and emancipation led to increasing opportunities for crime, and especially unfeminine forms of crime such as violence. She added that the link between emancipation and violence in women was proven by the rise in the tide of recorded female crime. Adler stated, "How else can we understand the female (or for that matter the male) offender except in the context of the social role? The mother becomes the child beater, the shopper the shoplifter, and the sex object the prostitute." Adler (1975) maintained that as the social and economic disparity between females and males decreased, female criminality would increase. She also believed that as social roles became similar, the types of crimes in which women would be found would be more similar to those of men. Adler reflected:

> Women are no longer indentured to the kitchens, baby carriages, or bedrooms of America. . . . [A]llowed their freedom for the first time, women . . . by the tens of thousands—have chosen to desert those kitchens and plunge exuberantly into the formerly all-male quarters of the working world . . . in the family that women are demanding equal opportunity in fields of legitimate endeavor, a similar number of determined women are forcing their way into the world of major crime. (1975, pp. 12–13)

Her correlation between increased emancipation and increased crime has been criticized widely because crime has not increased proportionately to emancipation.

Simon (1975) also focused largely on the influence of socioeconomic variables of women's criminality. She believed that changing rates in female crime (increases) are not to be attributed to differences in biology or psychological makeup but to differences in opportunities. She, too, theorized that as women increased their participation in the labor force, the scope and opportunity for criminal behavior would increase. Klein (1973) also postulated that criminal behavior and illegal activities were a viable economic alternative for economically deprived women. Rans (1978) supported this view. She attributes the increase in arrest for Part II crimes to the economic conditions of modern women. She emphasizes that the contemporary women offenders are faced with great demands to support themselves and their households, that they are often unemployed and responsible for children. Rans (1978) exhorts researchers to pay attention to the flux of changing economic conditions on arrest rates—e.g., inflation, unemployment, widening income gap, and increased female heads of households.

THE NATURE OF JUVENILE CRIME

In the United States, children from 7 to 18 traditionally are seen in the juvenile court after arrest. They are charged as delinquents rather than criminals. The term *delinquency* varies from one jurisdiction to another and generally is either an act that would be criminal in an adult or a status offense. A status offense is an act on the part of a juvenile that would not be considered a crime by an adult, such as running away from home, incorrigibility, curfew violation, or truancy. Generally, these delinquent acts are the types of behavior for which most young girls are arrested and charged. The traditional function of the juvenile court is to protect, treat, and rehabilitate adolescents. It is under the rubric of protection that most adolescent girls are arrested.

The juvenile statutes long have been thought to discriminate against adolescent offenders through overly vague and broad statutes and the maternalistic desire to protect, treat, and rehabilitate. Until recently, many states had juvenile laws on the books that contained higher age limits for girls—i.e., the age of majority or the age at which a youngster could remain under the jurisdiction of the juvenile court. That meant a girl could be charged with an offense that would not be an offense for an adult or for a male of the same age. For example, running away from home would be considered a delinquent offense for a late adolescent girl, but a boy of the same age would no longer fall under the jurisdiction of the juvenile court. In addition, a girl who was incarcerated for the same offense as a boy might have to remain in the juvenile correction institution for a longer period of time. In some states, for example, a 12-year-old female could be held in a correctional facility until she was 21 (Chesney-Lind, 1977).

ADULT WOMEN OFFENDERS

Although violent crime among women offenders has earned the most media attention, the vast majority of these offenders are arrested for victimless crimes—promiscuity and prostitution are the primary discriminatory legal offenses applied against the adult female. In contrast, very few men are arrested or jailed for being "Johns." In large urban areas, convicted prostitutes in jails constitute in excess of 50% of the female population (Haft, 1974). As noted earlier, women are next most likely to be incarcerated for Class II offenses—larceny or shoplifting is considered a female crime. However, men in large numbers shoplift.

In England and Wales, for every year from 1972 to 1982, some 200 women were convicted or questioned for robbery, while the numbers of men convicted of robbery rose over the same period from 2,500 to 4,300.

Compare these numbers with convictions for shoplifting. For shoplifting, in England in 1982, there were 48,000 convictions of males as compared with 32,000 for females. Thus, large numbers of men were convicted of what is considered only a woman's crime. Mehew (1977) suggested that shoplifting was one activity in which women's opportunities to commit crime were greater than any other, since shopping is a legitimate and indeed the central public activity for women. However, in a more recent and methodologically more exact study, Buckel and Farrington found that "men are proportionately twice as likely to shoplift as women." Moreover, men stole about five times as many items as did women, and these items were of considerably greater value. It may be that store security police are more on the lookout for women.

When women commit crimes of violence, they rarely are committed against strangers. Violent crimes are more likely to be committed against members of the family—infants, children, spouses, lovers. A recent explanation of violence in the family suggests that women become violent in the family when they perceive no other solutions to overwhelming psychological or social problems. For example, while mental health professionals may perceive a ready solution to a crisis of a battered wife, the battered wife herself may have tried social agencies, police, family, and friends for support and sustenance and found them unhelpful or no longer willing to help. She may perceive violence as the only available realistic solution to her dilemma.

THE PROFILE OF THE FEMALE OFFENDER

The most typical female offender is likely to be a young girl or young woman, first offender charged with shoplifting. Although the FBI's *Uniform Crime Reports* provides yearly arrest figures, the report does little to describe an actual profile of the women who are arrested and incarcerated. Single case studies are not of much help.

Glick and Neto (1977) completed an extensive survey of women in jails and prisons. They conducted the most comprehensive examination of women's correctional programs reported in many decades. The sample of 14 states encompasses states populated by approximately 52% of the female population age 13 and over in the United States. Their national sampling includes the states that contain approximately 52% of the female population age 18 and over in the United States and accounts for 66% of all women in U.S. jails and prisons. These sample states are representative of the total incarcerated female population in the nation. The investigators observed that imprisoned female offenders generally are young, between 18 and 29 years of age, with a median age of 24. They also note, as do others, that female felons tend to be single yet are mothers, have lower IQs, have had less formal and informal education than the average woman, and possess few work skills. Their prior work histories are in low-status jobs, usually service-related occupations. They are most likely to be from unstable or broken homes marred by alcohol and drugs, mental illness, and physical and sexual abuse. They are predominantly not white, but rather black or Hispanic.

CRIMINAL HISTORY. At least 50% of the women in Glick and Neto's (1977) studies had other family members who were incarcerated. Fifty-six percent reported friends who had been imprisoned or in jail. Forty-three percent of the female offenders themselves had been arrested for juvenile offenses and usually had been convicted of status offenses. Forty-nine percent of the total group had been arrested for the first time between 18 and 24 years of age.

ECONOMIC STATUS. A cycle of poverty was described by the vast majority of incarcerated women. Their income was obtained from marginal work, or a spouse, a lover, or welfare. Welfare was a subsistence existence slightly above the poverty level. Even the women who worked did so at low-paying jobs, and at least half the inmates who had worked earned less than $60 per week at the time of incarceration.

WOMEN'S PRISONS

Visitors to women's prisons usually are impressed by their campuslike atmosphere. In fact, such prisons typically are called campuses, just as some children's mental hospitals are called schools. Geographically, most women's prisons are located far from urban areas, in country settings. The tall brick fences, concrete walls, gun towers, and barbed wire typical of men's prisons are not present (Simon, 1975). The female inmate's quarters often have more privacy than the single rooms or cells of men. Women usually are permitted to wear street clothing and to decorate their rooms. However, the pleasant facade can be deceiving.

Women's prisons are described as more punitive (Giallombardo, 1966; Mann, 1984; Sobel 1982). The vast majority of women officers reflect the rural background from which they come. They also are poorly trained and most often are white females rather than members of the minority groups that constitute the prison population. The officers expect women to obey, to conform to their rules, some of which are unrealistic and not adaptive to community living. The prison officers are described as becoming the "inmate's parents" and taking control over her life (Burkhardt, 1976).

Interaction with officers and other inmates does not foster coping and social skills. Few women's prisons have provisions allowing female offenders to have their children live with them. Some have nurseries where infants can stay for varying lengths of time (McGowan & Blumenthal, 1976), but such facilities are rare. In areas where public transportation is not available, a woman may serve her entire sentence without seeing her children or family. In fact, some prisons prohibit visits of children under 16 years of age.

Because there are fewer women prisoners, as compared with men, institutional size seems to be smaller. As a result of this, there are fewer programs for institutionalized women. Women's prisons often do not have services designed to facilitate reentry into the community (Glick & Neto, 1977; Simon, 1975). Vocational programs are conventional and train women for traditional jobs in domestic work or cosmetology. Vocational programs, educational programs, and job assignments at women's prisons do not compare with those at men's prisons.

Medical services often also do not compare. Since the institution is small, medical aid is generally on a part-time basis and sporadic. Most frequent medical problems of incarcerated women reported by medical staff are gynecological, nervous anxiety, headaches, and pain. The most frequent chronic illnesses noted are diabetes, hypertension, epilepsy, drug addiction, and alcoholism. Medication is the most frequent treatment. In the Glick and Neto (1977) sample, 42 of the 53 institutions reported frequent dispensing of pain medication to inmates, followed closely by tranquilizers and psychotropic drugs. In many cases, medication is used as a panacea or an agent of social control. Other therapeutic techniques rarely are available.

Mental health treatment is almost nonexistent, despite the high instances of mental health problems (Benedek, 1985; Glick & Neto, 1977; Mann, 1984). Those psychologists and psychiatrists who work in prison programs report repeated conflicts between professional and treatment staff and custodial and nonprofessional personnel. Such conflicts discourage women professionals from working in the correctional system.

An increasing number of suits on behalf of women inmates are demanding equal correctional facilities. In a report prepared by the staff of the U.S. General Accounting Office, recommendations were made that would provide separate and equal treatment for women. Those recommendations included (a) shared facilities—coeducational correctional institutions for men and women that could share available resources; (b) community corrections as an alternative to incarceration or transitional facilities out of the correctional system, an approach that would facilitate contact between women and their families, increase sentencing alternatives, and offer more education and training opportunities; and (c) joint ventures among federal, state, and local levels to promote and utilize incarceration facilities. With more joint ventures, the population would be larger and the cost per inmate would be less for private industry, allowing private concerns either inside the institution or through contracts to provide products and services for women.

Recidivism

We continue to know little about female behavior over time, particularly recidivism. In reviewing official crime data, self-report data, or victimization data, it would appear that females commit less crime over time and less serious crime than males (Hindelang, 1981). Some authors believe that women released from correctional programs incur lower recidivism rates than males (Warren & Rosenbaum, 1986). They suggest that although women produce delinquent children, they themselves are unlikely to be processed again by the criminal justice system and returned to prison. Their hypothesis is supported by data found in parole records of some states. Such data reflect a 50% return to prison rates for males and only about a 10% return rate for females (Spencer & Beracochea, 1972).

Warren and Rosenbaum (1986) have looked at the criminal careers of female offenders and reported criminal dimensions of persistence, duration of offense behavior, crime specialization, and an escalation of seriousness over sequential career periods. They studied a group of women admitted to the California Youth Authority (CYA) between 1961 and 1969, through three time periods: from first recorded offense to the CYA commitment, from commitment to favorable or unfavorable discharge from CYA, and from CYA discharge to April of 1981. They were able to analyze the career paths of 159 juvenile offenders and were surprised to find that "(1) A large majority of our follow-up sample had arrests continuing into adulthood; (2) A large proportion had many arrests; (3) A very large percentage had arrests of moderate severity and almost half had arrests of high severity; (4) 85% had been convicted again, and 60% had been incarcerated."

They comment that this adult picture seemed all the more surprising when they noted that two-thirds of the young women were brought into the CYA for status conditions only. Interestingly enough, the seriousness of the adult offenses of the juvenile offenders also was unexpected. Forty-nine percent had been incarcerated for property offenses, but approximately half the women were arrested for offenses such as attempted robbery, delivery of narcotics, selling narcotics, assault to commit a felony, child abuse, child abandonment, attempted murder, robbery, and threatening with a weapon—crimes that were rated at a high level of severity. These authors also note that in the third period, i.e., the post-CYA commitment, there was some clear and consistent evidence of escalation of seriousness of the criminal offense. They closed their study by remarking: "The fact that our findings were surprising is worthy of note. It reinforces the idea that we know little about what happens to women offenders. The findings clearly point to the need for more longitudinal research."

CONCLUSIONS

As in the past, assumptions about female criminality and its etiology, treatment, and prognosis persist with little basis in empirical evidence and research literature. Despite the proliferation in the late 1970s of literature about female criminality, the statements have been for the most part anecdotal and not statistical. There is little real knowledge about the interaction of nature and nurture, of genes and environment, the development and history of the female delinquent. The literature focuses for the most part on the single sensational female criminal, the murderer, the terrorist. In addition, our rehabilitation efforts and our treatment of women offenders still remain primitive and elementary. Despite the often repeated expressed need for special jails and prisons, hospitals and health facilities, few specialized facilities exist, and there does not seem to be any movement to improve conditions for imprisoned females.

REFERENCES

Adler, F. (1975). *Sisters in crime.* New York: McGraw-Hill.
Benedek, E. (1985). Premenstrual syndrome: A new defense. In J. Gold (Ed.), *The psychiatric implications of menstruation.* Washington, DC: American Psychiatric Press.
Burkhardt, K. (1976). *Women in prison.* New York: Popular Library.
Chesney-Lind, M. (1977). Judicial paternalism and the female status offender. *Crime and Delinquency, 23,* 121–130.
Crites, L. (Ed.). (1976). *The female offender.* Lexington, MA: D. C. Heath.
Dalton, K. (1980). Cyclic criminal acts in premenstrual syndrome. *Lancet,* 1070–1071.
Giallombardo, R. (1966). *Society of women.* New York: Wiley.
Glick, R. M., & Netto, V. (1977). *National study of women's correctional programs* (National Institute of Law Enforcement and Criminal Justice, LEAA). Washington, DC: U.S. Government Printing Office.
Haft, M. (1974). Women in prison: Discriminatory practices and some legal solutions. *Clearing House Review, 8,* 1–6.
Hahn, N. F. (1980). Too dumb to know better: Cacogenic family studies and the criminology of women. *Criminology, 18*(1), 3–25.
Hindelang, M. J. (1981). Variations in sex-race-age-specific incidents rates of offending. *American Sociological Review, 45,* 461–474.
Holtzman, E., and Newman, B. (1984). *PMS: Symptoms of an unsound defense.* The Compleat Lawyer, 8, 9–11, 54.
Horney, J. (1978). Menstrual cycles in criminal responsibility. *Law and Human Behavior, 2*(1), 25–36.

Klein, D. (1973). The etiology of female crime: A review of the literature. *Issues in Criminology, 8,* 3–30.

Lombroso, C., & Ferrero, G. (1916). *The female offender.* New York: Appleton.

Mann, C. R. (1984). Race and the sentencing of female felons: A field study. *International Journal of Women's Studies, 7*(2), 160–172.

McGowan, B. G., & Blumenthal, K. L. (1976). Children of women prisoners: A forgotten minority. In L. Crites (Ed.), *The female offender.* Lexington, MA: D. C. Heath.

Pollak, O. (1950). *The criminality of women.* Philadelphia: University of Pennsylvania Press.

Rans, L. (1978). Women's crime: Much ado about. . . ? *Federal Probation, 42,* 45–49.

Report to the Nation on Crime and Justice. (1980). Bureau of Justice Statistics, Rockville, MD.

Simon, R. J. (1975). *Women and crime.* Lexington, MA: D. C. Heath.

Sobel, S. B. (1982). Difficulties experienced by women in prison. *Psychology of Women Quarterly, 7*(2), 107–117.

Spencer, C., & Beracochea, J. E. (1972). *Recividism among women parolees.* Sacramento: Department of Corrections Research Publication.

Sutherland, E. H., & Cressey, D. R. (1966). *Principles of criminology.* Philadelphia: J. P. Lippincott.

Thomas, W. I. (1907). *Sex and society.* Boston: Little, Brown.

Thomas, W. I. (1923). *The unadjusted girl.* Boston: Little, Brown.

Warren, M. Q., & Rosenbaum, J. L. (1986). Criminal careers of female offenders. *Criminal Justice and Behavior, 13,* 393–416.

Weisheit, R. A. (1984). Women and crime: Issues and perspectives. *Sex Roles, 11.*

Chapter 12

Battered Women

JANICE HUTCHINSON

"If a guy hit you once, he'll hit you again. Leave!" This is the advice my mother gave when I was a child. The battered women with whom I have met echo this sentiment. It is, they say, the single most important thing for a female to know about battering. Even so, there are many aspects of battering that must be addressed. This chapter will reveal a collage of information regarding battering of females: definition, epidemiology, history, sex roles assignments, characteristics of battered women and batterers, the wide range of injuries, roles of health professionals and law enforcement agencies, conflicts that battered women have about leaving, and solutions through prevention and treatment. Several case vignettes illustrate some of these issues.

HISTORY

The high rate of assaults against women and the high rate of non-reporting by women may imply a certain social/cultural acceptance. In fact, current attitudes regarding such battering find their roots in legal, religious, and cultural legacies that defined sex roles and created a marital hierarchy of male dominance and female submission. The word *family* is derived from the Latin *familia*, meaning the absolute possession of slaves by a single individual. The Roman emperor Romulus provided the first law of marriage in 753 B.C. He proclaimed that married women were "to conform themselves entirely to the temper of their husbands and the husbands to rule their wives as necessary and inseparable possessions" (Dobash & Dobash, 1977–1978). Single life was discouraged,

JANICE HUTCHINSON • District of Columbia Department of Mental Health, Washington, D.C. 20009.

so almost all young people married. Ownership and total control of property were placed with the man; the wife was legally obligated to obey the husband. Laws reflecting a double standard were created to enforce this system. Cato, the censor, declared in the 5th century B.C., "If you catch your wife in adultery, you could put her to death with impunity, she, on her part, would not dare to touch you with her finger; and it is not right that she should" (Dobash & Dobash, 1977–1978).

Subsequently, a new religious group, the "Christians" appeared. Some members of that group taught partial and misapplied scriptures throughout the centuries that have promulgated women-battering. They were vigorous and clear in their support for patriarchy and a marital hierarchy that made the man "the shepherd," and the women and children "the flock." Scripture as interpreted by these zealots is replete with passages taken out of context that empower men and subjugate women: "For the man is not of the woman; but the woman of the man" (I Cor. 11:8). ". . . wives be in subjugation to your husbands" (I Peter 3:1). ". . . the head of the woman is the man" (I Corinthians 11:3). "But I suffer not a woman to teach or to usurp authority of man, but to be in silence" (I Timothy 2:12). "And if they will learn anything, let them ask their husbands at home" (I Corinthians 14:34–35).

These passages form the foundation of support for patriarchal marriage. These teachings were later codified into law. The laws of chastisement dominated the Middle Ages. Once married, the man owned his wife and all of her goods. Men in Spain, Italy, France, and England had license to chastise disobedient wives by public flogging, exile, or death. By English Common Law, a married woman had no civil rights, enjoyed no separate legal status, and was chattel of the husband.

The new American colonies adopted English law. In 1824 the supreme court of Mississippi gave husbands the right to chastise wives. A court in North Carolina ruled in 1864 that the state should not interfere in cases of domestic chastisement and that the parties should be left to themselves unless permanent injury or excessive violence occurred. Wife-beating finally became illegal in Alabama and Massachusetts in 1871. In 1891 courts determined this to be a morally incorrect practice, and by 1910 all but eleven states permitted divorce on the grounds of cruelty.

For cultural and political reasons the family has been regarded as a sacred institution, representing domestic tranquillity. The *Journal of Marriage and the Family* contained no indexed references to violence from its first publication in 1939 through 1969 (O'Brien, 1971). Child abuse, murder, incest, rape, and spousal abuse were nonevents. Violent acts between family members were considered a private affair, if not a legitimate norm. The Lou Harris poll of October 1968 revealed that one-fifth of the 1,176 Americans interviewed throughout the United States approved of slapping a spouse on appropriate occasions. In spite of the long history of the battering of woman and the extent of the problem, the first book that focused on the subject (Pizzey, 1974) was published only fairly recently.

Although the written law has changed, the spirit of the earlier law remains. The author Alani (1976) wrote that on some occasions "wives . . . deserved to be beaten." Patriarchy and its attitudes toward female and male roles are pervasive and persistent pieces of the current social fabric. They form the basis for the carryover of women-battering from the pre-Christian years to the late 20th century.

DEFINITIONS AND DEMOGRAPHICS

Battering refers to assaultive behavior between adults in an intimate and usually a cohabitating relationship. There are four forms of battering: physical, sexual, and psychological, and destruction of important personal items. Physical battering includes hitting, choking, burning, hair pulling, shooting, stabbing. Sexual battering is forced sexual activity, unwanted pinching of genitals and breasts. Threats to personal safety, control of a victim's activities, and attacks on self-esteem denote psychological battering. Some abusers destroy the victim's favorite and important personal goods, including property and pets.

All forms of battering occur without concern for the victim, to show power and control, and tend to increase in severity and frequency over time.

Wife was once defined as "a woman: formerly in a general sense; in later use restricted to a woman of humble rank or of low employment, especially in the sale of some commodity" (the *Compact Edition of the Oxford English Dictionary*, 1971). More recently, *wife* has been defined as a "woman joined in marriage to a man" (The *Random House Dictionary of the English Language*, 1987).

Wife-battering is no respecter of class. A popular myth is that marital violence occurs more commonly among lower-income persons and in "minority ghettoes." These groups are highly represented in public health statistics because they often seek service from public health agencies. Middle-class and nonminority persons are more likely to seek assistance through personal physicians, attorneys, and others. The Bard (1971) study showed that the number of wife abuse cases was approximately the same in the black working-class 30th Precinct of West Harlem as in the white upper middle class of Norwalk, Connecticut (Bard, 1971; Johnson, 1975). The two communities had nearly equal populations. The experiences of Charlotte Fedders, as detailed in her book, *Shattered Dreams* (Elliott & Fedders, 1987), has brought a new focus to family violence among the middle class. According to the 1968 Harris poll, 25% of college-educated people and 16% of those with 8 years of schooling or less approved of a husband's slapping the wife. Twenty-five percent of blacks, 20% of whites, 16% of females, and 25% of males approved of a husband's slapping the wife (Stark & McElroy, 1970).

Epidemiology

Because of the closeted nature of the offense, the real incidence of woman-battering is unknown. In testimony presented to the New York state legislature in April 1977, Langley (1977) estimated that there are 28 million battered women in the United States. Straus (1978) and Walker (1979) assert that approximately one-half of all married women in the United States have been physically abused by husbands. In major urban areas, 75 to 95% of complaints are filed by women (Martin, 1981).

According to FBI estimates, a woman is battered every 18 seconds. Stark, Flitcraft, and Frazier, (1979) reported that 54% of the identified battered women were beaten by their husbands, 34% by boyfriends, and the remainder by sons or other relatives. In 1986, 1,510 women were killed by spouses, ex-spouses, or boyfriends.

In a report of a Department of Justice's National Crime Survey, Klaus and Rand (1984) noted that 91% of spousal abuse crimes involved abuse of a woman by a husband or ex-husband. Twenty-five percent of the victims were abused at least three times in the 6 months preceding the survey.

Researchers continue to identify a relationship between spouse abuse and child abuse (the American Human Association, 1976; Gayford, 1975; Hilberman & Munson, 1977–1978). Battered women often express concern over the impact of the battering on the lives of their children. Studies reveal a high incidence of somatic and psychological sequelae among the children exposed to battering (Hilberman & Munson, 1977–1978). Impaired concentration and difficulty with schoolwork was common. Boys often develop disruptive behavior. Girls become withdrawn, passive, and clinging; they learn quickly that they cannot control or influence what happens to them.

A.B. is a 28-year-old suburban homemaker and mother of two children: a 9-year-old girl and a boy, age 4. She gave the following history in a group therapy session:

> I left my husband two weeks ago. We were married for ten years. At first, things were not so bad. I had a good job with the government, but he didn't want me to work outside. He said a woman's job was to work and clean in the home. He didn't want me to have any friends, and always wanted to

know where I was and treated me like I was a child. He could never admit he was wrong. He used to say "marriage is a dictatorship and you ain't got no dic(k)." I left him several times, but I always came back. He would apologize and, besides, I felt guilty about breaking up the family unit. But I got tired of the beatings; got tired of being treated like a dog.

I never saw beatings when I was a kid. I didn't want my kids to act like what they saw. My son is beginning to act like his father—demanding his dinner and telling his sister to do as he says. She is passive. I had to get them out of there. You stay because people blame you if things are not right . . . they call you a failure. I finally built up my own confidence, and I am gone for good. He says he'll get some treatment. Good for him. But I'm not going back.

TIME, PLACE, AND ONSET

Assault against women usually occurs in the home (Dobash & Dobash, 1979; Gelles, 1972). The most frequently cited times generally coincide with the evening meal and after work hours.

The abusiveness is usually preceded by verbal disagreements that are related to child care, sex, housework, and money. Most women experience at least two attacks a week. Attacks are relatively brief (15 minutes or less) or may continue for hours. Self-defense is infrequent (Dobash & Dobash, 1979). Regardless of the size of either spouse, the man is usually the stronger of the two.

FAMILY BACKGROUND

Many abused women have lived in violent families as children (Gayford, 1975; Scott, 1974) and left home at an early age to escape violent, jealous, and seductive fathers (Hilberman & Munson, 1977–1978).

C.D., a 32-year-old mother of three children, spoke about some of these issues in a group therapy session.

I was with him for four years. I left on Wednesday. We had a fight and he nearly killed me. I'm looking for a job now. I have a B.A. in English and was working as a legal secretary. The father of my two youngest children also beat me. I don't know how I got with these men. My dad sexually abused me when I was a kid . . . I'm not going back.

CHARACTERISTICS OF ABUSERS

Abusive men have been found to have common characteristics. Many were abused in childhood or gave histories of parental violence (Fleming, 1979; Hanks & Rosenbaum, 1977). They tend to experience themselves as weak and powerless. The commission of violent acts seems to give them a sense of strength and control (Fleming, 1979). Self-esteem is low, and they may disavow all responsibility for an attack, instead blaming the wife.

Elbow (1977) suggested that abusive men fall into one of four categories: the controller, the defender, the approval seeker, and the incorporator. The controller must control others to defend against losing control himself. The defender needs his wife to depend on him so that he can feel strong. Poor self-esteem is the basis for the violent acts of the approval seeker. He needs reaffirmation from others, especially his wife. The incorporator needs to have the strength of another to make himself feel complete, so he clings to his mate.

Hilberman and Munson (1977–1978) found that extreme jealousy was reported in 57 of the 60 abusive marriages that they studied. These men created an atmosphere of isolation for their wives, discouraging personal friendships and labeling the wives' friends as lesbians or trash. Several investigators (Gayford, 1975; Hilberman & Munson, 1977–1978; Scott, 1974) report that abusive husbands frequently accuse their wives of infidelity.

These men do not necessarily appear violent. Many abused women indicate that their husbands can be charming and pleasant, especially in public. Yet implicit in their description is the fact that they must also be aggressive. Aggressiveness in this society is compatible with masculinity and is therefore tolerated and desirable. Battered wives have reported that after the husband attacks them, he often wishes to have sex with them. The battering and the desire for sex are nearly synonymous. It reflects the man's sense of impotence, lack of control, and poor self-esteem that is relieved only with the assertion of physical strength. The phallus is like the fist—asserting control and forcing submission.

LIVING WITH ABUSE

What is the life of a woman with one of these assaulting men? Often, the victim sees herself as isolated from others. Extended family members, who might well serve as allies, are likely to be miles and miles away (Scott, 1974). Even if family members, or friends, are close by, a distance might be created by the battered woman's sense of shame. Not unlike some rape victims, battered women feel responsible for the violence. They may feel that there is something wrong with them and/or that they deserved to be beaten (Hirsch, 1981). Low self-esteem is likely to be an underlying characteristic. Of course, repeated assaults (physical or verbal) are bound to undermine any level of self-esteem or self-confidence. Any sense of independence that the battered woman may have experienced becomes sharply diminished, if not totally destroyed.

Some of the aforementioned characteristics might lead some clinicians to label a woman as masochistic. Scott (1974) suggests that caution be taken in making such a connection "for many of the alternative explanations are not easily appreciated—covert threats to her or the children, inability to find alternative housing or support, isolation" (p. 437). However, it is reasonable to suspect a masochistic element if there are no such barriers that would prevent escape.

EMOTIONAL AND PHYSICAL EFFECTS

Individual and/or multiple assaults produce multiple injuries—physical and psychological. Some women are strangled to unconsciousness. Sexual assault is a common part of the physical assault.

Rounsaville and Weissman (1978) reported that 19% of the abused women receive traumas that resulted in serious injury to the head, 5% have lacerations requiring sutures, and 62% have contusions and soft tissue injuries. Most likely sites of injury are the head and neck, but no part of the body is spared. About 40% of all female homicide victims are killed by husbands (Dobash & Dobash, 1977–1978, 1979). Psychiatric disorders, including self-abuse, and stress disorders are not uncommon sequelae of physical injury. One in 4 battered women attempted suicide at least once, 1 in 7 abused alcohol, 1 in 10 abused drugs, 1 in 7 was admitted to a state mental hospital, and 1 in 3 was referred for emergency psychiatric services/community health centers (Stark et al., 1979).

Hilberman and Munson (1977–1978) describe a stress-response syndrome among battered women not unlike the rape trauma syndrome. The greatest difference is that the former involves a pervasive and constant threat of assault. Battered women show agitation and anxiety bordering on panic.

Hopelessness, despair, guilt, shame, and powerlessness dominate their lives. Anger is generally controlled and self-directed in the form of suicidal behavior, depression, alcoholism, or self-mutilation. Forty percent of battered women in one study (Stark et al., 1979) attempted suicide the same day a battering incident occurred. Battered women were found to be nine times more likely to attempt suicide than nonbattered women. These are considered the last desperate defenses against homicidal rage.

Pregnancy seems to have a special role in relationship to abuse. A review of emergency room data is illustrative: Battered women were three times more likely than nonbattered to be pregnant at the time of injury (Stark et al., 1979). A New Hampshire survey revealed that one-fourth of families sampled reported violence during the pregnancy (Gelles, 1972). A 1979 Oregon study (Oregon Governor's Commission for Women, 1979) found that 40% of battered women said they were pregnant at the time of the beating. In another study (Helton, 1981) 35.3% of pregnant women interviewed identified themselves as battered. All but three had experienced battering prior to the pregnancy. Seven women reported an increase in battering with the pregnancy. The pattern of violence may change for some women during these 9 months. Women often say that the target for the beatings moves from the face and breasts to the abdomen, leading to an increased incidence of abortions and premature births.

Pregnancy seems to unleash the deepest and most intense anti-female feelings that the man has. Pregnancy, a clear definition of femaleness, is outside the possibility of male control. To that extent it is the ultimate threat to male dominance. So the woman is "barefoot and pregnant" and therefore more defenseless and vulnerable. Attacks directed to the breasts, vagina, and abdomen are random.

E.F., a 23-year-old woman with two children and 4 months pregnant, grew up in an environment studded with violence.

> I was gone 12 hours after the first hit. My boyfriend and I were doing OK when he came home one day and said he had arranged to sell the baby I was pregnant with. I told him that would only happen over my dead body. He got mad and beat me. He didn't even care that I was pregnant. After he hit me I prayed the Twenty-third Psalm. I turned to Jesus for help. I cried and packed my bags. I watched my mom leave my dad when I was seven. She was a prominent hard working woman in our hometown. Dad had damaged the car to prevent her from going to a meeting with the mayor. She told him no man could dominate her and her kids. I left with my kids and I'm not going back.

STAYING VERSUS LEAVING

The comment that most reflects the lack of understanding and confusion regarding battered women is the question "So why does she stay?"

In fact, women do leave. In the Dobash study (Dobash & Dobash, 1979) 88 to 96% of the women did leave at some time after an assault; some leave and return several times. They sought refuge with parents (44%), other relatives (25%), and friends (18%), or with neighbors (13%); some sought help at shelters.

Interviews with battered women indicate that nearly all are still in love with their mates in spite of the abuse. Women may engage in a pattern of staying, leaving, and returning over years. Reasons vary. Roy

(1977) identified two main factors: hope for change and no place to go. Fear of reprisal, children, economic dependence, fear of loneliness, and stigma of divorce were also listed in decreasing order. Women are more likely to seek outside intervention if the assaults become more frequent and severe, if there was not a pattern of conjugal violence in her family of origin, and if she is able to hold a job (Gelles, 1976).

Although women give many reasons for staying, fear seems to be the most common factor (Martin, 1981). This fear may lead to a pathological transference described by Ochberg (1980) as the Stockholm syndrome. The hostage begins to align himself/herself with the hostage-taker as a survival technique. The deep personal terror that the hostage feels leads to an adaptation to the situation; positive, dependent feelings develop toward the captor and negative feelings toward rescuers.

Religious and family expectations may keep a woman in a violent home. "A woman's duty," "till death do us part" are the rationales offered. Inadequate education, poor job skills, and unwillingness to go on welfare may make a woman reluctant to leave. A woman may believe that her marriage, her children, and her husband are all that she has or will have in life. She may need to feel wanted, if even by an abusing husband. If her self-esteem depends entirely on this, it will be hard for her to let go.

Walker (1979) suggests a rationale for the battered woman's psychological and physical paralysis in abusive relationships: These women are victims of learned helplessness. Repeated abuse leads to the development of an immobilizing sense of helplessness and powerlessness.

Sex-role socialization may support a woman's feelings of helplessness. It has been demonstrated that girls receive little feedback for good academic work, but greater positive feedback for social conformity. As girls learn these roles, they may also learn that they have little control over their lives no matter what they do. Self-determination is not possible; success must come through associations with men. So it is that battered women may learn that their responses do not make much difference.

G.H., a 31-year-old married woman with three children (ages 12, 6 and 18 months), spoke of her conflict about leaving her abusive mate.

> I was married for two years. My husband was on drugs and alcohol. A year ago, he pushed me down the stairs. I left him last year, but the family convinced me to go back because it was safer than staying away. I didn't know about him [about his assaultive, criminal behavior] prior to the marriage. He could be so charming and nice. He used to take care of his mother. My six-year-old son is in therapy now. He's in the hospital because he kicked the teacher. He also tried to commit suicide by running in front of moving cars. Now, I get counseling with him every week . . . I don't want to live with another man again.

THE INSTITUTIONAL RESPONSE

A frustrating aspect of the battered woman's experience consists of her seeking help from institutions that are ill-prepared and insensitive to her needs. The woman's sense of guilt and shame, her sense of privacy and respectability, and her belief that individuals and agencies will be unable and unwilling to help her influence her reluctance to seek help. Most of the assaults are unreported to police or medical agencies.

Police receive more calls for "family conflicts" than for all other categories of serious crimes, aggravated battery, and murder. Responses have often been passive, abusive, or nonexistent. Police receive little or no training in handling family disputes. They usually use "mediation" procedures—i.e., police separate the couple, discourage the wife from pressing charges, and walk the husband around to "cool off." Arrests are rarely made.

The effect of this nonarrest policy has become more apparent. In a study (Conflict Management: Analysis Resolution, 1973) of spousal homicides in Kansas City, Missouri, it was determined that police had been called at least once before the fatality occurred in 85% of the cases. In 50% of these cases they were called five times in the 2 years prior to the murder.

In response to the nonresponse of law enforcement officials, battered women are suing municipalities and their police departments. A recent landmark case in Connecticut represented the first time a battered woman (who had been partially paralyzed by the assaults) had been allowed to sue police in a federal court for failure to protect her from the husband. The court ruled that failure to protect a woman from a battering spouse constitutes sex discrimination, a violation of the Fourteenth Amendment. The court awarded her damages in excess of a million dollars. Similar cases are currently in litigation. The impact is notable. Several states, including Virginia, New York, Connecticut, and New Jersey, have adopted a proarrest policy if there is reason to believe an assault has occurred. Consequently, the number of family violence arrests have increased while the number of domestic homicides has declined.

Nonetheless, prosecution rates remain low. Battered women, terrified by the possibility of further abuse, fail to bring charges and bear witness, even after the husbands or boyfriends admit to their acts of violence.

Lawyers and prosecutors still hesitate to take these cases. They, too, prefer the mediation process to avoid the costs of litigation and to reduce the court workload; however, the primary reason not to take these cases is that women often drop the charges—they are too frightened of their mates to prosecute. Mediation is also thought to avoid hostility, to increase the ability of clients to negotiate solutions, and to avoid a long court process. However, as reported recently by the U.S. Commission on Civil Rights (1982), mediation has been found to be an ineffective remedy for wife abuse. This process places "the parties on equal footing . . . fails to punish assailants for their crimes . . . implies that victims share responsibility for the illegal conduct . . . requires them to modify their own behavior in exchange for the assailant's promises not to commit further crimes."

The Minneapolis Police Department conducted a study to determine which response (arrest, mediation, separation) to domestic disturbance calls was most effective in stopping future assault (Sherman & Berk, 1983). In cases where there was a separation of the parties for 8 hours, violence recurred in 24% of cases; in cases in which mediation occurred, violence returned in 17%; when an arrest was made, violence recurred in 10%. A study of a community-based mediation program in Brooklyn revealed that mediation between those in intimate relationships was four times more likely to dissolve than agreements between persons in nonintimate relationships. Domestic violence cases almost always involve intimate relationships, so mediation does not appear to be a good choice.

The first persons to see a battered woman in a medical setting are usually emergency room physicians. Their ability to recognize and treat the results of physical injury is undisputed, yet their ability to identify assault as the source of the injury remains questionable. Striking observations were made in a review of 481 medical records of women who sought emergency services (Stark, et al., 1979). According to the methodology used, emergency room physicians had identified 1 out of 35 patients as battered. Yet the reviewers found 1 in 4 was more accurate. Physicians noted that 1 injury out of 20 resulted from domestic abuse; review indicated that 1 out of 4 was more accurate. Battering was 10 times more frequent than physicians noted.

Physicians tended to give battered patients pseudopsychiatric labels: patient with multiple vague medical complaints" or "multiple symptomatology with psychosomatic overlay" or, simply, "neurotic" and "hypochondriacal." One in 4 battered women left the ER with one of these diagnoses, as opposed to 1 in 50 nonbattered women. One in 4 suspected battered women left the ER with prescriptions for pain killers and/or minor tranquilizers. Abused women do not always tell physicians the etiology of their injuries, nor do physicians always ask. The hurried, impersonal pace of the emergency room milieu does not sup-

port detailed history taking or history giving. Physicians are often uncomfortable with, and unconscious of, nonphysiological bases for illness
in their patients.

THERAPEUTIC INTERVENTION

Wife-battering is a problem of the present time and times past. Is
there no solution? Because wife-battering is so persistent and so pervasive, approaches to stopping the violence must be encompassing and
widespread. Solutions lie in prevention and treatment, in the responses
of the battered woman and the battering man, in the teachings of parents, and in the actions of the community and its institutions.

Woods (1965) has identified five essential tasks that the assaulted
woman must accomplish either on her own or with the assistance of
others: (1) learning that she does not deserve to be beaten, (2) identifying clearly the person who is responsible for the abuse—the person who
is assaulting her, (3) reflecting upon her role in the relationship with no
implication that she provoked the attack, (4) becoming aware of the
reasons why she remains in the relationship, (5) getting in touch with
her own reactions, especially the anger and the stress.

Anyone who interfaces with a battered woman should help her
develop a "safe plan," a plan to keep her and her children safe until she
can decide on a more permanent course of action. Safe plans might
include identification of all possible escape routes, removing weapons,
alerting a neighbor to a signal that would mean an attack is occurring
and police should be called, avoiding being trapped in the kitchen or
any room where there might be weapons, identification of a safe place
(e.g., a friend's home, relatives' home, a shelter), hiding money, gathering of important documents (e.g., birth certificate, bank account number, checks) in one place, teaching children to leave the scene of violence
and call for help. If an attack occurs and there is no way out, feigning a
seizure or a faint may stop the attack.

Later, if the woman decides to leave, there must be family and/or
friends available to her. The woman who leaves a battering situation is
often angry, depressed and resentful. She may present as abusive or
abrasive and emotionally depleted. Making an emotional connection to
another person will help reassure her and reduce her sense of isolation.
She must be helped to face the world outside of the home, often with no
money, shelter, or job. But she must learn eventually to trust herself and
her ability to succeed in a life outside of the home. She must be helped to
a brighter, happier sense of self.

Helping the battered woman means also helping the battering offender. The best thing anyone can do for a battering man is to stop him. He is out of control. There are an indeterminate number of programs in the United States designed to help battering men. One of the oldest in EMERGE, a men's counseling service on domestic violence. Its goal is to help men develop a self-image that does not require violence to support it. Some programs focus on "reconciliation," attempting to change sex-role stereotypes that contribute to man's tendency to control woman. Other programs use a theme-centered approach, exploring unresolved masculine issues and projecting positive images of personal growth, nurturance, intimacy, and nonviolence through thematic discussions. Many of these programs maintain close ties to battered women's shelters.

Parents can intervene early in the lives of their children to prevent battering. They can begin by modeling nonviolent behavior, resolving family problems in nonviolent ways. Father and mothers can raise each child, boy or girl, to have a positive sense of self, rather than raising them according to sex-role stereotypes. Children should be raised with respect for their individual skills and live in families that create self-esteem and self-confidence in their children. Parents must begin to teach their sons that striking a woman is an intolerable act, unless there is a situation that threatens his life. A daughter must be made aware of the early warning signs of abuse in a young man: Notice how he expresses frustration and anger, notice whether he blames others when angry or frustrated, learn about his attitudes toward women and children and his feelings about how families should operate. It would be in her interest to determine if he is able to listen to the opinions and feelings of others, especially women, and if he is jealous and possessive; also, if he requires his girlfriends to abandon their friendships and families. Excessive drinking and/or use of drugs should also be considered as an early warning sign.

Community support is essential in both prevention and treatment. Victim advocate projects provide acute assistance. They may give emergency help, provide liaison services, transport a woman to helpful agencies or shelters, and provide information on police, prosecution, and courts. Other projects will find housing, help the woman keep her job, assist in child care and shopping, providing protection, support, and solace to the woman in transition.

Locations and phone numbers of shelters are often kept confidential to protect the women from further assaults. Women can reside in these refuge homes for a period of several days to several months. Services provided include legal aid for assisting with issues of separation and divorce and warrants; social services to help obtain financial assistance, housing, food stamps, and day care; rehab programs for job training, employment counseling, and local educational opportunities; medical assistance for both medical and mental health care for themselves and their children. The biggest problem with shelters now is that there are too few. The need for shelters is lessened when family, friends, and neighbors come to the support of the abused women in the ways described above.

Community agencies, as well as individuals, must also begin to help redefine femininity and masculinity and concepts of sex roles. Masculinity should not mean the ability to have power and/or control over another. Relationships between men and women should be between equals and not according to a hierarchy.

The medical community can learn to identify and assist the battered woman in a variety of ways. Emergency room (ER) physicians, especially, must be able to respond since they are often the first physician contact. The protocol developed by Engels and Warshaw (1988) should be made available to ER staffs. The protocol advises physicians to have a high index of suspicion when (a) injuries are old and inadequately explained, (b) there are old and new fractures, (c) there are repeated visits with increasingly worse injuries, (d) there is child abuse or a pregnant woman miscarries. Physicians are encouraged to explore the possibility of abuse, in a nonjudgmental manner, in the course of obtaining the history and performing the physical examination. Appropriate referrals (shelter, social services, mental health counseling) should be made. In some states physicians are required to notify law enforcement agencies when a person appears for treatment secondary to assault.

Legal and law enforcement agencies could act to change the face of abuse. Laws must be created to require police to allow for the arrest of a violent spouse. Protection from further abuse must be provided to the woman who wishes to press charges against the abuser. The criminal justice system should be improved and expanded to make offenders responsible for their actions through prosecution. Counseling and/or other diversionary programs for abusers should be a required part of the rehabilitative process.

The primary institutions of society, family, medicine, religion, and criminal justice must send a message that violence toward spouses will not be tolerated. Representatives of all service agencies must be sensitive to the impact that their own male-dominated systems have on women. The concept of a family must be redefined to connote "partnership instead of ownership." Only when women and men can respect themselves and each other will the family members and others realize their complete and total potential.

REFERENCES

Alani, A. (1976). The battered husband. *British Journal of Psychiatry, 129,* 96.

American Human Association, The. (1976). *National analysis of official abuse and neglect reporting.* Washington, DC: U.S. Government Printing Office.

Bard, M. (1971). The study and modification of intra-familial violence. In *The control of aggression and violence: Cognitive and psychological* (p. 154). New York: Academic Press.

Compact Edition of the Oxford English Dictionary, The. (1971). New York: Oxford University Press.

Conflict management: Analysis resolution. (1973). Kansas City, MO: Kansas City Police Department.

Dobash, R. E., & Dobash, R. P. (1977–1978). Wives: The "appropriate" victims of marital violence. *Victimology 2*(3–4), 426–442.

Dobash, R. E., & Dobash, R. P. (1979). *Violence against wives.* New York: Freed Press.

Elbow, M. (1977). Theoretical considerations of violent marriages. *Social Casework, 58,* 515–526.

Elliott, L., & Fedders, C. (1987). *Shattered dreams.* New York: Harper & Row.

Engels, B., & Warshaw, C. (1988). *Battered women hospital protocol.* Unpublished manuscript.

Fleming, J. B. (1979). *Stopping wife abuse: A guide to the emotional, psychological and legal implications for the abused woman and those helping her.* Garden City, NY: Doubleday.

Gayford, J. J. (1975). Battered wives. *Medical Science and the Law, 15,* 237–245.

Gelles, R. J. (1972). *The violent home: A study of physical aggression between husbands and wives.* Beverly Hills, CA: Sage.

Gelles, R. J. (1976). Abused wives, why do they stay? *Journal of Marriage and the Family, 38,* 659–668.

Guttentag, M., Salasin, S., & Belt, D. (1980). Afterword. In *The mental health of battered women.* New York: Academic Press.

Hanks, S. E., and Rosenbaum, P. C. (1977). Battered women: A study of women who live with violent, alcohol-abusing men. *American Journal of Orthopsychiatry, 47,* 291–306.

Helton, A. M. (1981). The pregnant battered woman. *Response, 9*(1), 22–23.

Hilberman, E., & Munson, M. (1977–1978). Sixty battered women. *Victimology, 2*(3–4), (460–471).

Hirsch, M. F. (1981). To love, cherish and batter. In *Women and violence.* New York: Van Nostrand Reinhold.

Johnson, S. (1975). What about battered women? *Majority Report,* February 8, p. 4.

Klaus, P., & Rand, M. R. (1984, April). *Family violence* (Special Report, p. 3). Washington, DC: U.S. Department of Justice—Bureau of Justice Statistics.

Langley, R. (1977, April). *Wife beating: The silent crisis.* Testimony before the New York State Legislature.

Martin, D. (1981). *Battered wives.* (Rev. updated, p. 13). San Francisco: Volcano Press.

Meier, J. (1987, May). Battered justice. *Washington Monthly,* 37–45.

O'Brien, J. E. (1971). Violence in divorce-prone families. *Journal of Marriage and the Family,* 22(4), 692–698.

Ochberg, F. M. (1980). Victims of terrorism. *Journal of Clinical Psychiatry, 41,* 73–74.

Oregon Governor's Commission for Women. (1979, September). *Domestic violence in Oregon.*

Pizzey, E. (1974). *Scream quietly or the neighbors will hear.* London: IF Books.

Random House Dictionary of the English Language, The. (1987). New York: Random House.

Rounsaville, B., Weissman, M. M. (1978). Battered women: A medical problem requiring protection. *International Journal of Psychiatry in Medicine, 8,* 191–202.

Roy, M. (1977). *Battered women: A psychosocial study of domestic violence.* New York: Van Nostrand Reinhold.

Scott, P. D. (1974). Battered wives. *British Journal of Psychiatry, 125,* 433–441.

Stark, E., Flitcraft, A., & Frazier, W. (1979). Medicine and patriarchal violence: The social construction of a private event. *International Journal of Health Services, 3.*

Stark, R., & McElroy, J., III. (1970). Middle class violence. *Psychology Today, November,* 30–31.

Straus, M. A. (1977–1978). Wifebeating: How common and why? *Victimology: An International Journal* 2(3/4): 443–458.

U.S. Commission on Civil Rights. (1982). *Under the rule of thumb: Battered women and the administration of justice 96.* Washington, DC: U.S. Government Printing Office.

Walker, L. (1979). *The battered woman.* New York: Harper & Row.

Woods, F. (1981). *Living without violence.* Fayetville, Ark.: Project for Victims of Domestic Violence.

Chapter 13

Homeless Mentally Ill Women: A Special Population

Leona L. Bachrach

Introduction

Homeless mentally ill women clearly constitute what the President's Commission on Mental Health (1978) in the Carter years termed a "special population"—a subpopulation of American citizens who experience extraordinary and often unremitting barriers to care. Indeed, several areas of "specialness" converge to affect the access of homeless mentally ill women to needed services.

This chapter, a conceptual analysis of homeless mentally ill women as a unique service population, explores the interactive impact of gender, mental illness, and homelessness as barriers to care. More specifically, it analyzes the characteristics of this target population—women who are both undomiciled and disaffiliated, and who also fit the diagnostic and other criteria for chronic mental illness—by moving down a ladder of abstraction from the most general to the most specific. It discusses, in turn, the circumstances of homeless people in general, homeless people who have chronic mental illnesses, homeless women, and, finally, homeless mentally ill women.

This chapter thus responds to a largely unexplored area in studies of homelessness and particularly studies of the homeless mentally ill. Although a rapidly growing body of literature on these topics is emerging in the United States (Bachrach, 1984a), that literature concentrates primarily on men (Bachrach, 1988). Very few professional contributions even acknowledge gender differences within the homeless mentally ill

Leona L. Bachrach • Maryland Psychiatric Research Center, University of Maryland School of Medicine, Cantonsville, Maryland 21228.

population, and fewer still focus on homeless mentally ill women's special circumstances. However, studies of homeless mentally ill women are remarkably consistent in their reiteration of several basic themes: that these women are being evicted and displaced in increasing numbers all over the United States; that their meager personal resources are inadequate to sustain them; that their homelessness is somehow more "invisible" than that of men; that for virtually all of them, ready access to adequate health care, including mental health and supportive services, is a basic life necessity; and that most of them encounter severe barriers of various kinds as they seek access to those services.

HOMELESSNESS IN AMERICA

Several major observations may be made about the homeless population of the United States. A first observation concerns the fact that homelessness is a very difficult concept to define (Bachrach, 1984a, 1984b) and is so imprecise that it is not unusual for researchers and service providers to engage in heated debates about its dimensions and characteristics. Might a cardboard box, a reed hut, or an automobile reasonably be construed as a home? Might it be so construed under benign climatic conditions such as those that prevail in southern California? Indeed, is a simple lack of shelter by itself sufficient to render an individual homeless, or must other conditions be present as well?

In response to this confusion, some advocacy groups in Great Britain have attempted to clarify the definition of homelessness by introducing the concept of "houselessness." To these advocates, the term *houseless* implies only a simple lack of physical residence. But the term *homeless* is reserved for conditions of more generalized deprivation, and it implies disaffiliation as well (Bailey, 1977).

The notion of disaffiliation—that is, an absence of affiliative attachments and supportive social relationships—is exceedingly important in the definition of homelessness. It implies that homeless people, in addition to having no residence, also somehow lack the skills and the resources to move out of their circumstances (Segal & Baumohl, 1980). It suggests that their lives have become stalled and hopeless.

Homeless people may be found in many different places, if one knows how and where to look for them. They may be found on the streets, in the middle of streets, in cars, under cars, in parks, in libraries, in subways, in jails, and in general hospital emergency rooms. They also may be found in state mental hospitals, not necessarily because they need to be there in a clinical sense but because there is frequently no other accommodation available to them.

Thus, the homeless population is a very diverse one that consists of a variety of subgroups. Many routes—many combinations of events—

dispose people toward homelessness. In addition, homelessness exists in all regions of the country, among people of all ages and ethnic origins.

In the United States the prevalence of physical illness and physical debility is very marked in the homeless population. In addition to alcohol and other substance abuse, trauma, accidents, burns, respiratory infections, tuberculosis, cardiovascular disease, leg ulcers, cellulitis, acute gastrointestinal disease, seizure disorders, and insect infestations are common (Brickner, 1985).

The homeless population appears to be undergoing extensive demographic changes. Generally speaking, it is growing younger, and its patterns of morbidity, as well as its geography, appear to be changing. Whereas in earlier decades the homeless population consisted largely of middle-aged alcoholics living in inner-city slum districts, today's homeless population contains growing numbers of younger individuals who are geographically dispersed (Bachrach, 1984a).

This changing demography may be at least partially explained by the fact that the homeless population is being saturated with increasing numbers of economically distressed individuals—people who often are referred to as the "new poor" (Harrington, 1984). These are individuals who have lost their jobs and generally are down and out (Kerr, 1986; McCarthy, 1986). Because they are victims of poverty, they often cannot afford low-cost housing, even when it is available—and it often is not. And with what has been called the growing "feminization of poverty" during the 1980s (Bassuk, 1986; O'Connor, 1986; Stein, 1986), increasing numbers of impoverished single women, often together with their dependent children, are becoming a significant element in the homeless population.

CONSIDERATIONS OF TIME AND SPACE

The new demography of the homeless also is related to certain considerations of time and space. There are three separate kinds of mobility that may characterize people in today's homeless population (Bachrach, 1987a).

There is, first, movement into and out of the homeless population. Homelessness may be quite temporary, or it may be a more or less permanent circumstance. Several research reports now distinguish between permanent street people and the episodically homeless (Arce, Tadlock, Vergare, & Shapiro, 1983; Roth, Bean, Lust, & Saveanu, 1985), who move into and out of the homeless population—sometimes many times over.

The second type of mobility affecting the homeless concerns diurnal or seasonal movement within relatively small and well-defined geographic areas. Some homeless people live more or less continuously in one place. Other homeless people, while they may remain essentially in the same neighborhood, tend to branch out as shelters or other services become available to them, or as their specific needs for subsistence and health care shift. Some shelters impose stringent time limits on the number of days that a person is allowed to remain in residence and thus contribute to this type of mobility.

The third kind of mobility that affects homeless people is transiency—that is, mobility over wide geographic areas. Although many homeless people are relatively stationary, some of them—the exact proportion varies from place to place—move within and between the various regions of the country. The precise correlates of these gross migration patterns are not known, but there is little question that they prevail. They most likely are reinforced, perhaps even precipitated, by certain informal practices. For example, there are reports of homeless individuals who are recruited into migrant labor streams and then transported over considerable distances to migrant labor camps. After their work is finished, these individuals then are released to wander in the areas to which they were taken (Henry, 1983; Herman, 1979; Moore, 1985). There also is a practice known as "Greyhound therapy"—providing homeless people with one-way bus tickets out of town (Cordes, 1984; Shipp, 1985; van Winkle, 1980)—that almost certainly also contributes to these gross migration patterns.

Because the issue of transiency among the homeless has become somewhat politicized in recent years (Bachrach, 1987a), its influence should be considered in perspective. Not all communities experience transiency to the same degree. Communities actually vary substantially in the extent to which they attract geographically mobile homeless individuals; even *within* some communities, there are some observable differences.

Beyond this, few hard statistics concerning transiency in the homeless population are available. However, even if such numbers did exist, they probably would not begin to tell the whole story. There is reason to believe that many of the sickest members of the population are characterized by the greatest geographic mobility—so that, even when these people seem to be in a distinct numerical minority, they should not be dismissed as being a negligible part of the homeless problem (Bachrach, 1987a). These transient homeless mentally ill individuals may well be the most persistent users of health, mental health, and social services—far beyond their numerical representation in the total population of homeless people within a given community.*

---

*These observations are borne out in the preliminary results of research that is currently being conducted on homeless individuals using general hospital psychiatric emergency

Agencies and governments at times either minimize or maximize geographic mobility among the homeless according to their own philosophies concerning entitlements, catchmenting, and the like. Accordingly, great care should be taken not to read too much, *or* too little, into observations about transiency in homeless populations.

THE HOMELESS MENTALLY ILL

A portion of the homeless population, however it is defined, legitimately may be described as chronically mentally ill. These members of the homeless population, who have been called the homeless mentally ill (Lamb, 1984), are not only undomiciled and disaffiliated; they also suffer from major mental disorders and show evidence of being severely and persistently mentally ill and disabled.

However, making psychiatric diagnoses within this population is often very difficult. Baxter and Hopper (1982), two New York City researchers, have written very persuasively that if some homeless individuals diagnosed with chronic mental illnesses could receive "several nights of sleep, an adequate diet, and warm social contact, some of their symptoms might subside"—an observation more recently supported by the epidemiological research of Koegel and Burnam (1987). Establishing the presence of psychopathology may be complicated when an individual is suffering extreme physical deprivation.

The homeless mentally ill population has become the subject of intense political controversy and territoriality in some quarters. Many advocates for the homeless perceive the acknowledgment of mental illness for some members of the population to be a denial of their economic and social problems—a way of blaming the victim (Alters, 1986), although there is no reason to think that mental illness and poverty are mutually exclusive.

In any case, making a distinction, either theoretical or clinical, between homeless individuals who have chronic mental illnesses and those who do not is in no way either pejorative or discriminatory. It is merely an effort to identify some of the parameters of homelessness, so that the unfortunate people who suffer from its consequences may be offered the most appropriate services and supports.

Inaccurate diagnoses of mental illness must be regarded as reflect-

services in Tucson, Arizona. The Tucson Homeless Mentally Ill Study, under the direction of Jose M. Santiago, M.D., Michael K. Berren, Ph.D., and Leona L. Bachrach, Ph.D., is sponsored by the Department of Psychiatry at the Kino Community Hospital in Tucson, Arizona. The observations also are supported in unpublished reports from Dr. Stephen Goldfinger at the San Francisco General Hospital. For related research, see Chafetz and Goldfinger (1984).

ing inadequacies in the state of the art, not as political statements. That is why Dr. William Breakey (personal communication, 1986) of Johns Hopkins University has said that a diagnosis is not an indictment; it is a working hypothesis that assists professionals who seek to prescribe relevant care for homeless individuals.

Deinstitutionalization is often a significant element in homelessness among the mentally ill—an element that varies according to one's definition of *deinstitutionalization*, since there is no standard definition of that term. However, a broad definition of that phenomenon subsumes more than the mere depopulation of state mental hospitals. It also includes certain other practices that discourage admissions to these hospitals (Bachrach, 1978).

The homeless mentally ill population actually illustrates both of these aspects of deinstitutionalization. It contains individuals who have been institutionalized in the past, often more than once; it also contains other individuals who *never* have been institutionalized. The difference between these groups is generally one of patients' ages, not one of degree of illness or level of disability.

Thus, it is a mistake to measure the prevalence of mental illness in a homeless population on the basis of how many people have ever been institutionalized, even though a number of studies have done so (Bachrach, 1984b). The important point about deinstitutionalization as it relates to the homeless mentally ill is that, despite its accomplishments, the movement often actually has served to promote a unique kind of eviction. There frequently is no available alternative to the state hospital for many mentally ill people, either because alternative residences simply do not exist in the community or else because the people who might use those residences are too disabled to live in them.

HOMELESS WOMEN

Too often, inferences about homeless women are based on observations of homeless men and do not consider the differential effects of gender-related circumstances within the target population. Perhaps this error is made because homeless women constitute a distinct numerical minority within the total homeless population. Several surveys have shown that in many communities women constitute only about 18 or 20% of the total homeless population (Brickner, 1985; City of Boston, 1983; Roth et al., 1985; United Way, 1984).

The correlates of women's homelessness, although in many ways similar to those for homeless men, appear to have somewhat different distributions. For example, homeless women less often appear to have problems with alcohol and other substances than homeless men (Barker,

1986; Lenehan, McInnes, O'Donnell, & Hennessey, 1985; McGerigle & Lauriat, 1983; Morse et al., 1985). And although homeless women and homeless men share many of the same physical illnesses, homeless women, because of a sex-related tendency toward varicose veins and venous insufficiency, often suffer from peripheral vascular disease and its consequences as well. It is not unusual for women who live on the streets to have massively swollen legs (Brickner, 1985). In addition, some homeless women have been reported to exhibit more severe psychopathology than homeless men (Crystal, 1984; Lenehan et al., 1985).

Homeless women and homeless men also appear to differ substantially in their demography and their treatment histories. Homeless women most likely are somewhat less transient than homeless men (McGerigle & Lauriat, 1983), and men generally seem to have longer durations of homelessness than women (Morse et al., 1985).*

These reported differences between homeless men and homeless women must, however, be interpreted cautiously, for a variety of extraneous factors may bias them. For example, homeless women often show great reluctance to respond to researchers' questions, possibly moreso than homeless men. McGerigle and Lauriat (1983) report that almost one-third of sheltered women contacted for a study of homelessness in the Boston area refused to answer some or all of the interviewers' questions, about twice the percentage of homeless men. This finding suggests that researchers must carefully establish valid confidence limits within which to interpret reports coming from homeless women.

Another source of bias is related to the relative inaccessibility of homeless women. Many of these women—again, apparently moreso than homeless men—somehow hide in places that are not known even to researchers (Teltsch, 1986; Wynne, 1985), meaning that the women who actually are interviewed may bear little resemblance to the total population of homeless women in a given community. Homeless women who are approached or counted by researchers usually are the ones who use shelters, soup kitchens, and other facilities and often are a highly selected population.

This selection may result from a variety of sources. For example, facilities for women may be in such short supply that certain subgroups of the population are not able to compete effectively for available space. Women may not use available facilities because of the violence and abuse that often are prevalent (McKay, 1986), or because of a real or perceived threat that they will be sent to a state hospital (Baxter & Hopper, 1982).

Thus, homeless women appear to be more discriminated against and less equitably served than homeless men (Bachrach, 1987b). Shelters

---

*This finding also is substantiated in the Tucson Homeless Mentally Ill Study.

and other facilities for women appear, in many communities, to be in even scarcer supply than are those for men. Beyond this, the house rules in these facilities tend to be very much more rigid than those existing in facilities for homeless men, so that women often are extruded and unwillingly find themselves on the streets.

An example of a practice euphemistically called "rotation," a practice enforced in many women's, but not men's, shelters in New York City, illustrates this point. A nun working in such a shelter provides an eloquent description: "You see, we only have beds here for twelve women and we let twelve more women sleep sitting up in chairs. But there are thousands of women out there—thousands who have no place to live. So many ladies come here for shelter that we can only let them stay for four days before we send them back on the streets. We call it "rotation." four days in, three days out. It's horrible, but we don't have much choice" (Kates, 1985).

Once they have become homeless, many women lead lives in which violence, uncertainty, fear, and stigma are part of their daily existence. Two investigators in Boston, McGerigle and Lauriat (1983), describe the circumstances of these women: "Becoming homeless—no longer having a place to rest in privacy, prepare one's food, care for one's children, and store one's goods—is perhaps the most profound privation imaginable in our society."

HOMELESS MENTALLY ILL WOMEN

The foregoing generalizations about the homeless in the United States, about the homeless mentally ill, and about homeless women converge in the population of homeless mentally ill women. Indeed, homeless mentally ill women constitute an extremely underserved and very special target population—a population that has been bombarded with scores of problems. Their multiple disabilities interact to make these women uniquely stigmatized, uniquely vulnerable, uniquely lacking in resources, and uniquely difficult to serve. More specifically, homeless mentally ill women, whether they live in shelters or on the streets, generally lead lives that are beyond the ability of most middle-class researchers to understand. A psychiatrist (Graves, 1985) who moonlighted in two women's shelters in Washington, D.C., while she completed her residency, describes this difficulty. She says that her work in those facilities was a "true transcultural experience," so that: "Entering the shelter was what it must have been like to enter an asylum at the turn of the century. Acutely psychotic and volatile women were shouting obscenities at the workers or other women who roamed the halls.

The odor was horrendous. But the irony of it was that this was 1985 in the capital of the richest nation on the earth."

Kates (1985), a journalist, in describing a facility for homeless mentally ill women in midtown Manhattan, writes that these women must surrender all their money and have their bags inspected before they may be admitted to the facility. They then are subjected to an "interrogation by a bored aide with a blank form in front of her" and "led down a corridor without explanation, handed a cup of foul-smelling 'shampoo' to kill lice, and ordered to take a shower." Finally, they are "forced to submit," without any explanation, to gynecological examination.

Thus, homeless mentally ill women typically endure a variety of disabling life circumstances that derive from many sources. Some of their disabilities are related to their mental disorders. Some of their disabilities are related to their homelessness. And some of their disabilities are related to gender-specific circumstances.

For example, we know that certain facilities for homeless individuals expect men to "earn their keep" by doing household chores. Those same facilities may treat women more like privileged guests who get waited on by the men—a matter of what one writer calls "ladies' privilege" (Strasser, 1978). On the surface, this differentiation may seem to make life easier for the women. However, reinforcing helplessness in this manner may actually limit chances for successful rehabilitation among the chronically mentally ill (Bachrach, 1987a).

The problems of pregnant homeless mentally ill women are particularly serious, and they serve to give new meaning to the familiar concept of "comprehensive services." The case of Nancy Hopper, reported to the *Boston Globe*, provides a specific and very troubling illustration (McLaughlin, 1984). Ms. Hopper, a 27-year-old homeless woman, bled to death in a seclusion room at a community mental health center. Her ruptured ectopic pregnancy had apparently gone undetected when she was admitted to the mental health center. Clearly, disabilities from many sources operated simultaneously for Ms. Hopper to complicate her life—and, ultimately, to precipitate her death.

Summary and Conclusions

This chapter has focused on the multiple and interactive disabilities of homeless mentally ill women by analyzing the unique position of these women in reference to other service populations. Four major observations were made about homelessness in general:

- Homelessness, which is difficult to define, generally refers to both an absence of shelter and a lack of affiliation.

- The homeless population is very diverse and consists of many subgroups.
- The prevalence of physical illness and physical debility in the homeless population is overwhelmingly high.
- The homeless population appears to be undergoing extensive demographic changes at the present time.

Four additional observations were made about the homeless mentally ill:

- It is often very difficult to make valid psychiatric diagnoses for members of the homeless population.
- There is frequently politically inspired resistance to acknowledging the relationship between chronic mental illness and homelessness.
- Making a distinction between homeless people who are mentally ill and those who are not is an important step in sorting out some of the many variables that characterize homeless people.
- Deinstitutionalization, broadly defined, is often a significant factor contributing to homelessness among chronically mentally ill individuals.

Four observations also were made about homeless women:

- Homeless women apparently constitute a numerical minority within the total homeless population.
- Because homeless women differ appreciably from homeless men in a variety of ways, it is not advisable to make generalizations about homeless women that are based on observations of homeless men.
- Because of their general invisibility and their reluctance to respond to researchers, it is not advisable to generalize about all homeless women on the basis of observations of facility-based subpopulations.
- Homeless women appear to be more discriminated against and less equitably served than homeless men.

Finally, only one overarching observation was made about homeless mentally ill women: Multiple disabilities from many different sources converge and interact to make these women uniquely stigmatized, uniquely vulnerable, uniquely lacking in resources, and uniquely difficult to serve.

These several observations lend depth and perspective to the subject of homeless mentally ill women and permit some general hypotheses concerning other special populations. First, we may hypothesize that special populations often are invisible. Not only may they be hidden physically from the service system, but the uniqueness of their service needs also may be masked. Accordingly, case-finding efforts, to say nothing of service delivery strategies, might be very creative. If planners go to the same old places to find members of special populations—if they try to identify patients in the same old ways—they may miss these populations altogether.

We also may hypothesize that the multiple disabilities that typically affect special populations tend to be interactive to a degree that members of these populations have characteristics and problems that are unique. It follows that special efforts must be made to capture that uniqueness in research and service planning in order to enhance continuity and comprehensiveness in their care.

We may hypothesize further that society in general, and sometimes even clinicians and other service providers, often react to members of special populations in stereotypical ways. Not infrequently, such reactions take the form of unwarranted political polarization, which makes the members of special populations vulnerable to the vicissitudes of political controversy.

A specific instance of such polarization is provided in an event that occurred in Los Angeles County several years ago. Roman Catholic social workers were ordered to stop referring homeless women to a shelter operated by a nun who allegedly had a "proabortion position" (Shelter, 1985). Some individuals might question why the nun's position on the issue of abortion should deprive homeless women of shelter. However, the mere fact that such an order was issued suggests that decisions affecting special populations may have relatively little to do with the populations' service needs and a great deal to do with the needs of special interest groups.

In conclusion, we may observe that scientists and clinicians who identify members of special populations, or who make recommendations about mental health services for these individuals, must check their assumptions and their methods constantly. Standardized techniques sometimes do more to confound than to enlighten when it comes to making generalizations about special populations. Members of these populations typically consist of people who have few advocates and few spokespersons. They are utterly dependent upon the professional community to get the facts straight.

REFERENCES

Alters, A. (1986). Roots of homelessness debated at conference. *Boston Globe*, March 28, p. 16.

Arce, A. A., Tadlock, M., Vergare, M. H., & Shapiro, S. H. (1983). A psychiatric profile of street people admitted to an emergency shelter. *Hospital and Community Psychiatry, 34,* 812–817.

Bachrach, L. L. (1978). A conceptual approach to deinstitutionalization. *Hospital and Community Psychiatry, 29,* 573–578.

Bachrach, L. L. (1984a). The homeless mentally ill and mental health services: An analytical review of the literature. In H. R. Lamb (Ed.), *The homeless mentally ill.* Washington, DC: American Psychiatric Press.

Bachrach, L. L. (1984b). Interpreting research on the homeless mentally ill. *Hospital and Community Psychiatry, 35,* 914–917.

Bachrach, L. L. (1987a). Geographic mobility and the homeless mentally ill. *Hospital and Community Psychiatry, 38,* 27–28.

Bachrach, L. L. (1987b). Homeless women: A context for health planning. *Milbank Quarterly, 65,* 371–396.

Bachrach, L. L. (1988). Chronically mentally ill women: An overview of service delivery issues. In L. L. Bachrach & C. C. Nadelson (Eds.), *Chronically mentally ill women* (pp. 3–17). Washington, DC: American Psychiatric Press.

Bailey, R. (1977). *The homeless and empty houses.* Middlesex, England: Penguin Books.

Barker, K. (1986). Street woman: Long day's journey into night. *Washington Post,* February 16, pp. A1, A11.

Bassuk, E. L. (1986). Homeless families: Single mothers and their children in Boston shelters. In E. L. Bassuk (Ed.), *The mental health needs of homeless persons.* New Directions for Mental Health Services No. 30. San Francisco: Jossey-Bass.

Baxter, E., & Hopper, K. (1982). The new mendicancy: Homeless in New York City. *American Journal of Orthopsychiatry, 52,* 393–408.

Brickner, P. W. (1985). Health issues in the care of the homeless. In P. W. Brickner, L. K. Scharer, & B. Conanan (Eds.), *Health care of homeless people.* New York: Springer.

Chafetz, L., & Goldfinger, S. (1984). Residential instability in a psychiatric emergency setting. *Psychiatric Quarterly, 56,* 20–34.

City of Boston Emergency Shelter Commission. (1983). *Seeing the obvious problem.* Boston: City of Boston.

Cordes, C. (1984). The plight of the homeless mentally ill. *APA Monitor,* February, pp. 1, 13.

Crystal, S. (1984). Homeless men and homeless women: The gender gap. *Urban and Social Change Review, 17* (Summer), 2–6.

Graves, M. (1985). Working with homeless women: A transcultural experience. *Spectrum* (Newsletter of the American Psychiatric Association/National Institute of Mental Health Fellows), November, pp. 3–6.

Harrington, M. (1984). *The new American poverty.* New York: Holt, Rinehart & Winston.

Henry, N. (1983). The long, hot wait for pickin' work. *Washington Post,* October 9, pp. A1, A16.

Herman, R. (1979). Some freed mental patients make it, some do not. *New York Times,* November 19, pp. 1, 4.

Kates, B. (1985). *Death of a shopping bag lady.* San Diego: Harcourt Brace Jovanovich.

Kerr, P. (1986). The new homelessness has its roots in economics. *New York Times,* March 16, p. E5.

Koegel, P., & Burnam, M. A. (1987). *Problems in the assessment of mental illness among the homeless: An empirical approach.* In M. J. Robertson & M. Greenblatt (Eds.), *Homelessness: The national perspective.* New York: Plenum Press.

Lamb, H. R. (Ed.). (1984). *The homeless mentally ill.* Washington, DC: American Psychiatric Press.

Lenehan, G. P., McInnes, B. N., O'Donnell, D., & Hennessey, M. (1985). A nurses' clinic for the homeless. *American Journal of Nursing,* November, 1237–1240.

McCarthy, C. (1986). The homeless: Bad policy, not bad luck. *Washington Post*, February 23, p. H2.

McGerigle, P., & Lauriat, A. S. (1983). *More than shelter: A community response to homelessness*. Boston: United Planning Corporation and Massachusetts Association for Mental Health.

McKay, P. (1986). My house is a lonely bed in a dreary D.C. shelter. *Washington Post*, February 16, pp. C1, C3.

McLaughlin, L. (1984). Mental health center death being probed. *Boston Globe*, December 11, p. 16.

Moore, M. (1985). Va. weighs migrant workers' plight. *Washington Post*, August 29, pp. A1, A21.

Morse, G., Shields, N. M., Hanneke, C. R., Caslyn, R. J., Burger, G. K., & Nelson, B. (1985). *Homeless people in St. Louis: A mental health program evaluation*. Jefferson City: Missouri Department of Mental Health.

O'Connor, J. (1986). Children bear brunt of homeless problems as families go wanting for shelter. *Psychiatric News*, May 20, pp. 20, 32.

President's Commission on Mental Health. (1978). *Report to the President*. Washington, DC: U.S. Government Printing Office.

Roth, D., Bean, J., Lust, N., & Saveanu, T. (1985). *Homelessness in Ohio: A study of people in need*. Columbus: Ohio Department of Mental Health.

Segal, S. P., & Baumohl, J. (1980). Engaging the disengaged: Proposals on madness and vagrancy. *Social Work, 25*, 358–365.

Shipp, E. R. (1985). Cities and states strive to meet winter needs of homeless. *New York Times*, December 25, p. 10.

Shelter is ruled off-limits. (1985). *Washington Post*, January 25, p. A8.

Stein, A. (1986). Children of poverty: Crisis in New York. *New York Times Magazine*, June 8, p. 3ff.

Strassner, J. (1978). Urban transient women. *American Journal of Nursing*, December, 2076–2079.

Teltsch, K. (1986). A haven for Boston's "invisible" women. *New York Times*, March 31, p. B7.

United Way of Greater Tucson. (1984). *1984 United Way homeless survey results*. Tucson, Arizona: Author.

van Winkle, W. A. (1980). Bedlam by the bay. *New West*, December 1, pp. 81–90.

Wynne, J. D. (1985). *Women on skid row: San Diego's invisible victims, 1984*. San Diego: County of San Diego Health Services.

PART V

Sexual Issues

Chapter 14

Homosexuality and Parenting

Martha J. Kirkpatrick

Homosexuality has long been considered antithetical to childrearing. We have held this conviction despite the wide acceptance, perhaps preference, for single women as teachers, governesses, and nurses and the welcome help from maiden aunts, bachelor uncles, and schoolmasters, many of whom may have been homosexual, at least in thought if not in deed. Although we have known for a long time that heterosexual males are by far the most frequent offenders in the sexual abuse of children, we continue to harass and discriminate against homosexual teachers of both sexes. Homosexuality has been deemed socially irresponsible at best, and, at worst, homosexual individuals have been considered likely to molest children and/or proselytize homosexuality.

A desire to avoid parental responsibility has even occasionally been cited as a motivation to become homosexual. Up until the last decade, homosexual parents were simply unheard of—and for good reason. A suspicion of homosexuality, even if unconfirmed, was sufficient to deprive a divorced mother of child custody and to deny visitation rights to a divorced father. Adoption or foster parenting by homosexuals was not considered appropriate. Further, revealing such proclivities to adoption agencies might result in job loss or other discriminatory actions against the applicant.

Historical Background

In the mid-1960s the homosexual community joined the waves of minority groups demanding equal protection and civil rights. In 1969 the gay liberation movement was born when the habitués of a gay bar,

---

Martha J. Kirkpatrick • Department of Psychiatry, University of California School of Medicine, Los Angeles, California 90024.

205

the Stonewall Inn in Greenwich Village, fought against a police raid. In addition, the rising political consciousness of women as a result of the women's movement and its ambivalent but declared support of lesbian issues gave mothers the courage to no longer deny or hide their sexual preference during custody proceedings.

Judicial interest shifted from the question of the presence of homosexual interests to the effect of the parent's homosexuality on the child. At least in some courts parental fitness had ceased to be discredited simply by the presence of homosexuality. In the early 1970s, a Michigan court (*Spence* v. *Durham*, 1973) awarded custody to a lesbian mother and her lover. According to the Lesbian Rights Advocates, a San Francisco based legal group, between 40–70% of cases involving lesbians fighting for custody of their children are won by the lesbian parent. The range reflects the experience in different areas of the country. In 1973 the American Psychiatric Association removed homosexuality from its diagnostic manual of disease categories. The American Psychological Association and the American Sociological Association made similar statements. In 1975 the governor of Pennsylvania issued an executive order directing all state agencies and departments to work toward ending discrimination against sexual minorities. About half of the states have begun similar efforts to decriminalize and end discrimination against homosexuals.

While these events have contributed to the courts' readiness to discount homosexuality itself as an issue in custody contests, many courts continue to place restrictions of association on the homosexual parent. These restrictions may prevent the homosexual parent from living with a partner of the same sex, or having the same-sex partner present when the child is present, or having the child in the home at all. Other restrictions of association may proscribe taking the child to any activity related to gay politics or gay community functions.

The judicial system has been hampered by a lack of published data on the effect of a parent's homosexuality on the child's development and by a lack of experienced expert witnesses. Homosexuality is assumed to mean not simply same-sex partners but a different life-style. No reports have confirmed or described this difference.

Before the liberation movements, researchers who wanted to collect relevant data had no way of identifying the population. Researchers who were homosexual themselves and might have had access to the gay world frequently avoided this area of research for fear of being identified or presumed to be homosexual. Highly functioning gay individuals were unavailable for study. The growing pride and political power of the gay community have changed this attitude by providing a source of self-esteem and community support. For the first time we can learn about this population in all its social diversity. Researchers are no longer limited to patient, prison, or organized gay groups for study populations.

The research, while just beginning, is accumulating new data that will prove essential to the courts in making custody decisions and to social agencies concerned with the placement of both homosexual and heterosexual children and the assignment of children to homosexuals as adoptive or foster parents. Such information is also invaluable to physicians asked to serve as expert witnesses or to give advice to homosexual parents. In addition to these specific uses, the data on homosexual parents throw light on many misconceptions and pose new questions about our vision of family life and its relationship to child development.

HOMOSEXUALS' INTEREST IN BEING PARENTS

ADOPTIVE OR FOSTER PARENTING. Some social agencies concerned with the adoption or placement of children have become aware of a population of single and coupled homosexual men and women wishing to be adoptive or foster parents. Some states openly or covertly use homosexual foster homes. California and Washington State have affirmative policies on the use of homosexual adoptive or foster homes, but these policies are vague and are primarily supported by nondiscrimination policies toward sexual minorities. The California Family and Children's Services indicated that in 1980 four gay homes were licensed to provide full-time foster care. A New Jersey survey found that most social agencies in various states reported no policy. Many reported a few instances of using gay homes, while others denied their use or that there were any homosexual homes in their community. Many social agencies said they were aware of homosexuals who had attempted to become adoptive or foster parents and whose efforts had been thwarted solely because of their sexual preferences. As of 1983 very few homosexual adoptions were on record: one in San Francisco by a gay male couple (a pediatrician and a minister) and one by a gay male minister in New York State. California's first single-parent adoption, about 20 years ago, was by a homosexual male. At this writing, there are no data on the success or problems that may result from these placements. The Lesbian Rights Project in San Francisco has begun an adoption project in response to many calls received each year from gay men and women wishing information and assistance in adopting children. For our purposes it is sufficient to note that there is a population of homosexual men and women who want to become adoptive or foster parents.

The movement toward non-discriminatory evaluation of gays as potential adoptive or foster parents received a severe setback in May of 1985. An openly gay male couple in Boston had been approved after investigation and participation in the foster parent training program by the Department of Social Service. Brothers 3½ and 2 were placed in their home in April. In May a sensationalized story in the *Boston Globe* about the placement prompted DSS to remove the children. Newspaper editorials demanding "normal" and "traditional" family placements resulted in Governor Dukakis's demand for a new policy. The new policy states children are to be placed in "traditional family settings . . . with relatives, or in families with married couples, preferably with parenting experience." Further, no placement with a unmarried couple or with a single person will be made "unless it can be clearly demonstrated that there is no traditional family setting available, or likely to be available." (Both New York and New Hampshire have considered similar policies. This policy, which places marital status ahead of all other considerations, was developed without significant input from professionals dealing with children. The Massachusetts Association for Mental Health, Massachusetts Human Services Coalition, Massachusetts Psychiatric Society, Massachusetts Psychological Association, and the National Association of Social Workers–Massachusetts Chapter cosponsored a forum on June 21, 1985 on "Foster Care Parenting and the Placement of Children with Gay Parents.") Forty professional organizations and agencies presented statements emphasizing that the best interests of the child are not *necessarily* met in "traditional" families and that the ability to parent is not determined by sexual orientation. (Despite the unprecedented unanimity of all these organizations, the policy was still in effect in January of 1986.)

A serious problem is locating suitable homes for gay teenagers who have run away or have been rejected from their own homes because of their homosexuality. William La Barr of Young and Gay, a New York homophile organization, estimates that on any given day in New York City there are as many as 2,000 gay children without homes. A 1980 survey of 90 child welfare workers, reported by the Bureau of Research of the New Jersey Division of Youth and Family Services, found that the great majority (80%) believe it was appropriate to place homosexual youths in homosexual homes. The welfare workers also reported a desire for additional training about issues these teenagers face.

NATURAL PARENTS. Recent studies of homosexual men and women have found that about 20% of the male sample and even more of the lesbian sample have been married. Bell and Weinberg's monumental 1978 study of approximately 600 homosexual men and approximately 300 homosexual women confirmed this 20% figure for the men and found that more than 30% of the women had been married. They reported that at least half of these marriages produced children. While we have no way of accurately computing the number of children with homosexual parents, the number is not as insignificant as we once believed.*

Cheri Pies, a licensed clinical social worker in San Francisco, runs a 6-week structured discussion program for lesbians who would like to become parents. She reports having seen 150 to 200 gay women and has also received calls from gay men requesting help in finding women who might coparent and/or bear their natural children.

In recent years unmarried women who want to become mothers have begun to arrange insemination and plan to rear their children alone. Fay Pannor, marriage and family counselor in Los Angeles, began the Alternative Parenting Network as a support system for women who want to bear the children of men who do not want marriage. The network now serves any unmarried woman who wants to have a baby. During less than 1 year of operation, 160 contacts were initiated. Pannor has estimated that at least 40% of these women were lesbians, which again confirms the substantial interest in parenting among gay women.

THE LIFE-STYLE OF HOMOSEXUAL PARENTS

Since the early 1970s, when the research population became visible, increasingly sophisticated studies have examined the life-styles of lesbian mothers (Goodman, 1973; Bryant, 1975; Lewin & Lyons, 1979; Lewin, 1981; Miller, Jacobson, & Bigner, 1981; Pagelow, 1980). A few studies (Bozett, 1981; Miller, 1979) have surveyed gay fathers. The results present a picture quite different from that which social mythology has led us to expect.

Whether observed in mothers' groups (Goodman, 1973), responding to questionnaires (Bryant, 1975), interviewed in their homes (Steirn, 1976; St. Marie, 1976), or interviewed in a comparative research study (Lewin, 1981; Lewin & Lyons, 1979), gay mothers were found to be remarkably similar to their heterosexual counterparts. While lesbian women generally tended to be better educated and economically better off than heterosexual women, lesbian mothers shared the less affluent, economically burdened position of most single mothers.† In our study (Kirkpatrick, Smith, & Roy, 1981) of the children of lesbian mothers, we

---

*Calculations of the number of lesbians with children range from Hoeffer's (1979) conservative estimate of 200,000 or 3% of the 6.6 million female heads to Martin and Lyon's (1972) suggested figure of 3 million or 30% of the estimated 10 million lesbians in the United States.

†Bryant's 1975 questionnaire survey of 185 self-identified lesbian mothers included data on education and employment. Compared with the statistics on the general female population, the lesbian group was better educated and more often professionally employed. Bell and Weinberg (1978) found that members of their white lesbian cohort were more likely to

controlled for the sex and age of the children, not for the mother's socioeconomic status or organizational affiliation. We found an unexpectedly similar diversity in both the subject and comparison groups, ranging from women who were financially independent to women who depended on welfare, from professionally trained women to high school dropouts; we also found a wide variety of living conditions in both groups. The majority of women had worked in traditionally female fields: education, nursing, and clerical.

Marital Histories

Even more surprising were the similarities in marital histories. We were confronted with our own prejudicial assumptions when we discovered that the marriages that produced both our subject and our comparison children were contracted at the same average age and usually for the same reason (namely, love of the husband and desire for marriage). Further, we found that the marriages of both groups had lasted the same average length of time—7 to 7½ years. These findings were corroborated by the Hotvedt study in the eastern and southern states and the Golombok British study.

Example 1. During college Sally N married a dental student. The couple had three children, two girls and a boy. Sally's husband had a good practice and the family moved a number of times, finally acquiring a large, comfortable home in an affluent suburb. Sally N felt increasingly lonely and distant from her preoccupied and isolated husband. She returned to school and earned a graduate degree. Although Sally derived pride and pleasure from her job, her life continued to feel "flat." She had a brief affair with a male neighbor but found no relief from the growing sense of inner desolation. She was aware of homosexual fantasies and occasional feelings for other women, which she put out of mind. After 18 years of marriage she found herself passionately involved with a woman her age whom she had met in a professional organization. She entered psychotherapy and, after 2 years of difficult work, separated from her husband.

Six years later, Sally N still found that her lesbian relationship provided the intimacy, warmth, and understanding she did not experience in her marriage. Sally N was able to remain in her home with her children, two of whom were in college. Her income reduced, she went to work full time. After several months of preparation with the children, her lover moved in, shared expenses, and participated in family events.

have completed college than were members of the white heterosexual cohort. There was no difference in educational history in their small black sample.

While the events, activities, and interests in her life have not changed since her lesbian relationship began, Sally N feels she is a more available mother now because of her feelings of fulfillment in her personal life, and the equal sharing of domestic responsibility with her partner.

EXAMPLE 2. Threatened by her father with detention in a juvenile hall or marriage to her high school lover, Myra P chose marriage at 17. She became pregnant and delivered a child by age 18. Her husband was unemployed and spent most of his time using drugs and attending rock concerts with his buddies. Myra finished high school and took a secretarial job. She spent her free time with girlfriends while her grandmother took care of her daughter.

Now in her late 20s, Myra has spent the last 5 years in a lesbian relationship with another mother of two small boys. Neither receives child support and the family income is marginal. Myra P is actively involved in several women's organizations and spends little time with her child, a situation that leads to fights with her disapproving partner. Family life is crowded, tense, and frustrating, although stable. Both of these marital situations were mirrored in stories told by divorced heterosexual mothers in our comparison group.

Both sets of mothers found their primary identity in their role as mother and complained of the same difficulties: money, housing, child care, and custody arrangements. Most mothers in both groups spent nonworking time with their children or were involved in child-centered and household activities. In both groups, we found that mothers who had live-in companions were more comfortable with their lives and provided richer family lives for their children. The age or sex of the partner, or type of relationship, sexual or nonsexual, did not seem to be relevant to the enriching and supportive effect of the partnership.

Our society's stereotype of lesbian couples has led us to expect a caricature of traditional male/female marriage roles. The authors of the previously mentioned studies commented on the lack of role-playing in their samples. We also found the responsibilities of lesbian couples divided on the basis of time and talent, not defined role. The nonmother partner functioned as an assistant mother, big sister, or aunt, but not an imitation father. In our study (Kirkpatrick, Smith, & Roy, 1981), we noted that children frequently reacted to the loss of the mother's lover with depression and a resurgence of reactions seen during the initial divorce of parents. Marriage and divorce statistics give us a means of approximating frequencies and durations of heterosexual commitments. We have no means of establishing the durability of lesbian relationships, nor do we know if lesbian mothers' relationships differ in duration from those of lesbians who have no children. Studies of lesbians that have included questions about the length of relations have been directed toward lesbians in their 20s. Those early relationships typically lasted 2 to 3 years. Studies in which older lesbians were included have documented that relationships of 20 years or more are not uncommon. The majority of lesbians have relatively stable, long-term relationships and place great value on being coupled (Peplau & Gordon, 1983). We do not yet know how the presence of children affects these relationships. The advent of children being born into established lesbian relationships requires new contracts regarding responsibilities and privileges of the nonbiological parent.

Support Systems of Lesbian Mothers

National statistics show that about half of divorced mothers are awarded child support and about half of these mothers receive regular payments. Lesbian mothers receive child support neither more nor less often than other divorced mothers. Some lesbian mothers are especially vulnerable to intimidation from ex-husbands who threaten to use their lesbianism to deprive them of custody unless they waive spousal support or lower child support payments.

In our study, while several mothers feared custody battles, the only contested case was a lesbian mother suing to establish paternity from a disinterested father. Both groups of mothers felt that continuing interest from the fathers was essential and beneficial to their children. In our study, lesbian mothers even more than the heterosexual mothers made efforts to provide adult male figures in their children's lives. Possibly the heterosexual mother assumed that a new marriage would provide a male figure for their children. A similar but even greater difference in favor of fathers attending to children of lesbian mothers was found in Golombok's British study.

In a study of support systems for lesbian and heterosexual single mothers, Lewin and Lyons discovered that both groups valued strong ties with kin. The lesbian community was not a significant source of support for lesbian mothers, perhaps no more than married couples' previous social system provides support for divorced heterosexual mothers. Although exposure of homosexuality strained family relations, parents and other relatives were the preferred source of emotional and practical support and provided the cushion during a crisis. Eighty-four percent of the lesbian mothers Lewin and Lyons interviewed said that most or all of their relatives know of their homosexuality. In some instances family ties were temporarily disrupted by the disclosure, but most families were able to restore their intimacy and mutual support.

One of the lesbian mothers in Lewin's study described her own mother's response: "Once in a while it will come up, and we'll talk about it. It's real painful for them. They don't want to hear it. So most of the time I don't talk about it. It's a very tight family and my mother says, 'We can't disown you. We can be really sad and unhappy about what you're doing and you are making a big mistake, but we love you and that's that.'"

Some heterosexual mothers and some lesbian mothers maintained close relationships with ex-husbands and continued to provide mutual support. Lewin and Lyons (1979) found that motherhood rather than sexual orientation provided the most salient feature in self-definition for both sets of mothers. Their life-style and support systems were built around their identity as mothers. Again belying the stereotypical expectation, lesbian mothers were not "driven by sex" or preoccupied with the sexual aspect of their lives. On the contrary, the sexual aspect of lesbian lives seems to be a preoccupation peculiar to the heterosexual society.

PARENTING ATTITUDES OF HOMOSEXUALS

Several recent studies (Hoeffer, 1979, 1981; Rees, 1979) have examined lesbian mothers and heterosexual mothers on specific parenting attitudes; the researchers have used a variety of instruments. Mucklow and Phelan (1979) examined 34 lesbian mothers and 47 heterosexual mothers on self-confidence, dominance, and nurturance. They found no significant differences in mean scores. Rees (1979) used the Parental Attitude Research Instrument and California Personality Inventory to compare 12 lesbian and 12 heterosexual single mothers. Again the results showed no significant difference in parenting style.

Hoeffer (1979, 1981) examined the mothers' influence on the children's acquisition of sex role and sex-role behaviors. She tested 20 lesbian and 20 single heterosexual mothers and their only or oldest children, who ranged in age from 6 to 9. The mother's encouragement of sex-role behavior was measured through the Toy Preference Test. Each mother was instructed to rate toys in order of preference for her child. Hoeffer also used a version of Fling and Manosevitz's Parental Interview, asking the mothers to describe gifts, activities they shared with their children, and methods of showing approval and disapproval. While heterosexual mothers showed a greater tendency to emphasize sexual dichotomy, both groups of mothers tended to encourage children to play with toys that were considered conventionally appropriate for their sex rather than opposite-sex toys. Both groups encouraged unisex toys more than sex-specific toys for both boys and girls. Both groups of mothers reported more involvement with daughters' play than with sons' play, a finding consistent with studies of two-parent families.

While our own study (Kirkpatrick, Smith, & Roy, 1981) was directed at evaluating the children, we spent 2 to 5 hours interviewing each mother and also conducted a home visit. Our unidentified prejudicial stereotypes were made obvious to us when we found we were surprised that the lesbian mothers most frequently supported feminine interests in girls and masculine interests in boys. The comments we heard most frequently in response to their hopes for their children's future were "I'd prefer my child were heterosexual. It's just a lot easier," or "I want my children to be whatever they want to be. I try to give my children the confidence to be themselves." No mother expressed a wish that her child be homosexual. We asked mothers if, and how, they had told their children about sexuality, and found considerable diversity, but we did not find difference on the basis of the mother's sexual orientation. About half of the lesbian mothers said their children knew about their sexual preference either because they openly discussed lesbian issues or because they had felt that honesty would promote trust and understanding in their children. Others felt the children would be confused and would not benefit by having such knowledge until they were older. A few felt that children would be better off never knowing. We found the child's views of the mother's relationship to be more a consequence of the child's developmental stage than of the mother's efforts at either disclosure or secrecy.

EXAMPLE 3. Eight-year-old Mary had been raised by her mother and her mother's lesbian lover almost since birth, although they had not lived together until Mary was about 2. Mary's mother and her lover were both political leaders in the gay community, frequently speaking in public forums and holding meetings in their home. Mary's mother assured me that her daughter knew all about lesbianism. Mary, however, told me coyly that her mother was going to marry a gay man who happened to be a close friend. This fantasy clearly had its source in Mary's developing heterosexual interests, which made use of this relationship for reinforcement.

Studies of lesbian mothers have shown that lesbians, like other mothers, organize their identity and life-style around motherhood. This common priority is reflected in the similarity of their primary concerns and activities. While parenting styles may vary, they seem to be relatively independent of sexual orientation. As Simon and Gagnon, reported in 1969, showed, the expression of feminity in the lesbian community resembles that in the heterosexual community and represents successful feminine socialization despite homosexual object choice.

Parenting interest and style appear to be more closely related to socialization than to object choice. The latter may be determined by earlier unconscious intrapsychic processes. The effects of feminine socialization can be detected in the responses to BEM's Sex Role Inventory (Bem, 1975). Several investigators (Hoeffer, 1981; Hotvedt, Green, & Mandel, 1979; Kirkpatrick, Smith, & Roy, 1981) have asked participants to complete this sex role inventory and have obtained curious results. They all found similar scores on femininity for both lesbian and heterosexual mothers.

Despite the similarity in femininity scores, Hoeffer pointed out that the lesbians had higher masculine scores and were more androgenous, while more heterosexual mothers scored as undifferentiated. If lower self-esteem and an undifferentiated "sex-role trait profile" are linked, as the literature suggests (Bem, 1975), these single heterosexual mothers may be at special risk for problems related to self-esteem.

CHILDREN WITH HOMOSEXUAL PARENTS

Before the publication of the most recent studies of children with a homosexual parent, it was assumed these children would be at risk for difficulties in sexual development, perhaps in overall psychological development, and would also be stigmatized by outsiders. Contrary data have resulted from a number of studies, although all of the studies have limitations and are far from providing complete understanding. Green (1978) reported on the results of interviews and play sessions with 21 children of homosexual parents involved in custody disputes. He found these children to be unremarkable when compared with children of heterosexual mothers.

In more carefully controlled studies (Hoeffer, 1979, 1981; Hotvedt et al., 1979; Kirkpatrick, Smith, & Roy, 1981; Rees, 1979) researchers matched children of lesbian and heterosexual mothers by age and sex and used a number of investigative instruments. For example, Hoeffer (1979) asked children between the ages of 6 and 9 to rate themselves on five male-valued traits (outgoing, adventuresome, never cries, strong, likes to be a leader) and five female-valued traits (aware of others' feelings, gentle, behaves, neat, quiet) on a 4-point scale for ideal and real self. The children were also asked to rate peers of the same sex. Hoeffer also measured sex-role behavior by Bock's Toy Preference Test. She found that the two groups of boys did not differ on sex-role traits or sex-role behavior; both groups also chose an androgynous sex-role trait profile as their ideal. The boys of lesbian mothers, however, rated themselves higher on two female-valued traits (awareness of others' feelings and gentleness) than did boys of heterosexual mothers. The two groups of girls did not differ on sex-role behavior. The girls of lesbian mothers rated themselves higher on two male-valued traits (adventuresome and likes to be a leader) than did girls of heterosexual mothers. Both groups of girls also chose an androgynous ideal.

Investigators have been unable to confirm that sexual confusion or pathology of any type is more frequent in children of lesbian mothers than in children of heterosexual mothers. None of the studies reviewed here has uncovered any sexual development differences in psychological tests, toy and activity preference, or reported interests and future wishes.

In our study (Kirkpatrick, Smith, & Roy, 1981) all of the children underwent a playroom evaluation by a child psychiatrist and testing by a child psychologist. These examiners were unable to distinguish children of homosexual parents from those of heterosexual parents. Each child was assigned a position on the Rutter scale according to the combined ratings of the psychiatrist and the psychologist. After categorizing the 40 children as severely disturbed, moderately disturbed, or minimally or not disturbed, we found similar numbers of each category in both groups. Among the severely disturbed children, the boys showed evidence of gender confusion, but the girls did not. One severely disturbed boy was from a lesbian family, the other was not. What they had in common was not their mothers' sexual orientation but a history of serious physiologic difficulties in early life.

EXAMPLE 4. Carl was the result of his mother's seventh attempt to carry a child. His mother hemorrhaged severely and spent most of her pregnancy in bed. Carl was born prematurely and was asthmatic until he was 5 years old. At 6 weeks he was discovered to have undescended testes. When Carl was 2, his physician attempted to pull down the testes by attaching rubber bands to Carl's thighs. Carl was terrified when a rubber band broke. When Carl was 5 years old he was found to have a bladder tumor that had been causing painful erections. The tumor and one testicle that had become malignant were surgically removed. After this surgery Carl became interested in playing dress-up in his mother's high heels and wig. When his mother began encouraging and participating in masculine activities with him (for example, working on a motorcycle, or fishing), Carl's feminine behavior disappeared.

When he began school, Carl was diagnosed as being hyperactive with serious learning problems and outbursts of violence. Now he attends a special school and therapy has been recommended. Carl's lesbian mother remains very devoted to his care, despite the difficulties and her minimal financial resources. It is hard to identify what part his mother's sexual orientation plays in his problems, if any.

We found approximately the same number of children from each group in the minimal or no disturbance category.

EXAMPLE 5. Six-year-old Janie had been conceived by artificial insemination performed by her mother's lesbian lover after her mother had tried several times to conceive through intercourse and an application for adoption had failed. Pregnancy and delivery were uneventful. The couple broke up when Janie was 3. Janie missed the lover and was mildly depressed and irritable while her mother went through a period of dating both men and women and had another pregnancy that ended in miscarriage. The friends and lovers of Janie's mother continued to be predominately homosexual. For the last year the mother and child have lived with a woman friend who is not a lover.

A winsome, comfortable child, Janie related well to both the male and female examiners. She indicated a close attachment to her maternal grandfather. Her mother told us that Janie had seen him only twice for brief periods, but she was able to make good use of this figure to complete her intrapsychic representation of parents of both sexes.

In the Golombok et al. study, only a very small number of children showed significant psychiatric problems. However, the proportion was substantially greater in the heterosexual single parent group (8 out of 35) than in the lesbian groups (2 out of 31). These investigators do not attempt an explanation for this finding. We believe it is noteworthy that while all of 27 of the heterosexual mothers were alone with their children, only 9 of the lesbian mothers were alone. The rest live with a lover or with 1 or 2 other adults. Thus the lesbian mothers were single only in terms of legal marital status and not in terms of child rearing setting. We have come to think of the presence or absence of another adult, especially one who is available to the child, as the most significant variable.

In summary, controlled studies with formal testing procedures suggest that the children of lesbians are not at risk for gender disorder or any specific pathology. There are, however, a number of caveats to be considered: None of these studies was longitudinal, nor have there been follow-up studies of the tested population. Tests for gender identity and object choice in prepubertal children are not definitive; the fluidity of character development phases, age-specific intrapsychic conflicts, and childhood fantasies makes efforts to prophesy future personality resolutions extremely difficult. For example, we found children with a history of cross-dressing who did not show evidence of gender confusion on one test but did on another. Finally, we have no follow-up studies of the adolescent or young adult population whose sexual identity would be tested more readily.

CLINICAL EXPERIENCE

Further suggestive evidence of specific pathology in these children comes from the rare reports of clinic population. Osman (1972) reported on family therapy with a lesbian couple and two sons, while Weeks, Derdeyn, and Langman (1975) reported on two cases of children of homosexuals. These therapists concluded that the parents' struggle with sexual conflict had an impact on their attitude and behavior toward their children but that these problems were not significantly different from those of heterosexual parents with sexual conflicts.

Javaid (1983) has provided a detailed account of an adolescent daughter's response to her parents' divorce and her mother's subsequent lesbian relationship. In therapy the girl, who had a twin brother, initially exhibited anxiety and somatization after the divorce. Later the girl walked in on her mother and a female lover. Soon after this experience the daughter had intercourse for the first time, followed by a pseudocyesis.

She continued to struggle with fears about her own sexual identity, but was relieved when her mother disclosed the sexual relationship with her lover. The daughter than experimented with homosexuality but returned to shallow relationships with boys for reassurance of her normalcy.

She felt abandoned by her father, who remarried and took her twin brother to live with him. Eventually the girl was able to express anger at her mother for depriving her of her father and was relieved at the mother's continuing love. She confused her need for nurturance from her mother with incestuous wishes and had another pseudocyesis.

Gradually the symbiotic tie began to dissolve, and the girl established a separate self with a heterosexual identity. Although the therapist did not provide the antecedent events in the girl's development that would help clarify the symbiotic tie to the mother, the struggle with differentiation appeared to be the girl's major difficulty.

It is impossible to know whether the girl's difficulty with separation-individuation is related to a similar struggle her mother may have undergone that was later manifested in a lesbian relationship. This clinical account magnifies the difficulties in adolescent individuation from parental images.

Hall (1978) and Lewis (1980) have reported the reactions of less disturbed children. Lewis interviewed a nonpatient group of 21 children from eight different lesbian families. The children confirmed the conclusions the researchers mentioned earlier that the breakup of the marriage was by far the most painful and upsetting event, much more upsetting than the disclosure of the mother's homosexual relationship. This revelation, however, was a source of shock, confusion, and pain to many children. She reported that the children's first reactions varied from "My God, you can't be one of those!" to pleasure that the "mother is more real now." She found that older boys showed initial hostility primarily aimed at the lover. These children were concerned about having a secret that made them feel different from their peers, and some questioned their own future sexuality. According to Lewis, the girls wondered if they, like their mothers, would change in later years, while boys struggled with bruised self-esteem and anger.

The children also reported relief from the parental battles and from the fear that their mother would be alone and would need their care. Some reacted by experimenting briefly with homosexuality; others exhibited maladaptive behavior, such as causing trouble to drive away the intruder, engaging in premature sexual activity, or becoming pregnant. The children tended to defend and protect the mother. Some, especially boys, reached out to their father and were able to establish a better relationship than they had had before their parents were divorced. The lover's arrival resembled the entry of a stepparent, but lacked the legal tie. Jealousies and resentments were less severe when the children were prepared and when the lover was willing to understand that the children's acceptance would take time. Many of these children had had some therapy at the time of the divorce, but most felt that family therapy was more helpful in maintaining or reestablishing good feelings toward other family members. Lewis concluded from her research that "the parent's sexual preference does not matter as much as the love, caring, and maturity of the adults and their efforts to help the children become self-reliant and self-assured."

DISCUSSION

Contrary to popular belief, many homosexuals want to become parents, and a significant number of children are currently living with lesbian mothers or are visiting gay fathers. The literature on gay fathers is very sparse, but a number of controlled studies and clinical reports have focused on lesbian mothers. Rather than being marked by a different life-style, lesbian mothers appear to be indistinguishable from single heterosexual mothers. Among both groups of women, motherhood is the single most salient feature of their personal identity, and their lives are organized around their children. Lesbian mothers may be somewhat more likely to support androgynous characteristics in both daughters and sons, but their expectations of their children's sexual development resemble those of heterosexual mothers. Lesbian mothers, at least as much as other single mothers, are concerned with supporting their children's relationships with their fathers and other men.

Our current testing tools do not reveal differences in the sexual, interpersonal, or social development of the children of homosexual parents. Parenting capacity does not appear to be a function of object choice. All of the children showed evidence of suffering because of marital conflicts and divorce. While the mother's disclosure of her homosexuality was not as upsetting as the divorce, many children were shocked, confused, hurt, embarrassed. Young children need to deny the meaning of the information; older children may be burdened by the secret or have concerns for their own sexual development, with an increased pressure to act out their heterosexuality for reassurance. As in all situations that necessitate a reorganization of family structure, family therapy may be helpful in confirming the continuity of the family, and in maintaining communication about these difficult issues.

Prior to these studies, both clinicians and courts assumed specific and serious consequences if a child were left in the care of a homosexual parent. Sexual confusion and high risk for homosexuality were expected. Although these fears have not been confirmed, we cannot assume that a parent's homosexuality has no effect on a child, only that the effects are variable in direction and extent, and there is specific or inevitable effect. Our research tools are clumsy, however, and important data are still missing. For example, only a few of the children in these studies were raised from birth by a mother who was in a lesbian relationship. Thus, these studies simply confirm our belief that both gender identity and sexual orientation are firmly established before the age of 5. Our understanding will be furthered by longitudinal studies of adolescents and young adults.

The currently available data lead us to reevaluate the importance of various parental characteristics necessary for responsible childbearing. Heterosexuality may not be as important as parental self-esteem, personal integrity, or the capacity to maintain consistent, loving relationships. Parents with supportive partners, regardless of their sex, are able to make better use of their own resources when responding to their children's needs. Modeling may not be as important to the development of sexual identity as parental support of the child's autonomy; such autonomy will allow the child to make use of many sex-appropriate models. Further study will shed light on these important developmental issues as well as provide expertise in the specific area of parenting by homosexual men and women.

REFERENCES

Bell, A., & Weinberg, M. (1978). *Homosexualities: A study of diversity among men and women.* New York: Simon & Schuster.
Bem, S. L. (1975). The measurement of psychological androgeny. *Journal of Consulting and Clinical Psychology, 42,* 155–162.
Bozett, F. (1981). Gayfathers: Evaluation of the gayfather identity. *American Journal of Orthopsychiatry, 5,* 552–559.

Bryant, B. (1975). *Lesbian mothers*. Unpublished master's thesis, School of Social Work, California State University.

Curran, D., & Parr, D. (1957). Homosexuality: An analysis of 100 male cases seen in private practice. *British Medical Journal, 5022*, 797–801.

Golombok, S., Spencer, A., & Rutter, M. (1983). Children in lesbian and single-parent households: Psychosexual and psychiatric appraisal. *Journal of Child Psychology and Psychiatry, 24*(4), 551–572.

Goodman, B. (1973). The lesbian mother. *American Journal of Orthopsychiatry, 43*, 283–284.

Green, R. (1978). Thirty-five children raised by homosexual or transsexual parents. *American Journal of Psychiatry, 135*, 692–697.

Hall, M. (1978). Lesbian families: Cultural and Clinical issues. *Social Work, 23, 5*, 380–385.

Hoeffer, B. (1979). *Lesbian and heterosexual single mothers' influence on their children's sex-role traits and behavior*. Paper presented at the Annual Meeting of the American Psychological Association, New York.

Hoeffer, B. (1981). Children's acquisition of sex-role behavior in lesbian mothers' families, *American Journal of Orthopsychiatry, 51*, 536–643.

Hotvedt, M., Green, R., & Mandel, J. (1979, September 4). *The lesbian parent: Comparison of heterosexual and homosexual mothers and children*. Paper presented at the Annual Meeting of the American Psychological Association, New York.

Javaid, G. (1983). Case report: The sexual development of the adolescent daughter of a homosexual mother. *Journal of the American Academy of Child Psychiatry, 1983, 22*, 196–201.

Kirkpatrick, M., & Smith, K., Roy, R. (1981). Lesbian mothers and their children: A comparative study. *American Journal of Orthopsychiatry, 51*, 545–551.

Lewin, E. (1981). Lesbianism and motherhood: Implications for child custody. *Human Organization, 40*, 6–14.

Lewin, E., & Lyons, T. (1979). *Lesbian and heterosexual mothers: Continuity and difference in family organization*. Paper presented at the Annual Meeting of the American Psychological Association, New York.

Lewis, K. (1980). Children of lesbians: Their point of view. *Social Work, 25*, 198–203.

Martin, D., & Lyon, P. (1972). *Lesbian women*. New York: Bantam.

Miller, B. (1979). Gay fathers and their children. *Family Coordinator, 28*, 544–552.

Miller, J. A., Jacobsen, R. B., & Bigner, J. J. (1981). The child's home environment for lesbian vs heterosexual mothers: A neglected area of research. *Journal of Homosexuality, 7*, 49–56.

Mucklow, B., & Phelan, G. (1979). Lesbian and traditional mothers' responses to adult response to child behavior and self concept. *Psychology Reporter, 44*(3), 880–882.

Osman, S. (1972). My stepfather is a she. *Family Process, 2*, 209–218.

Pagelow, M. (1980). Heterosexual and lesbian single mothers: A comparison of problems, coping, and solutions. *Journal of Homosexuality, 5*, 189–204.

Peplau, L., & Gordon, D. (1983). The intimate relationship of lesbians and gay men. In G. R. Allgeir & N. B. McCormick (Eds.), *Changing boundaries: Gender roles and sexual behavior*. Palo Alto: Mayfield.

Pies, C. (1985) *Considering Parenthood: A Workbook for Lesbians*. San Francisco: Spinsters, Inc.

Rees, R. L. (1979). A comparison of children of lesbian and single heterosexual mothers on three measures of socialization. *Dissertation Abstracts International*, Section B, 3418.

Saghir, M., & Robins, E. (1973). *Male and female homosexuality: A comprehensive investigation*. Baltimore: Williams and Wilkins.

Simon, W., & Gagnon, J. (1969). Femininity in the lesbian community. *Social Problems, 15*, 212–221.

Spence v. *Durham*. (1973). 198 SE, 2nd 537.

Steirn, C. (1976). *We are a family: An exploration of eight lesbian family units*. San Francisco: Lymar Associates.

St. Marie, D. (1976). *A descriptive study of lesbian mothers*. Unpublished master's thesis, School of Social Work, University of Hawaii.

Weeks, R., Derdeyn, A. P., & Langman, M. (1975). Two cases of children of homosexuals. *Child Psychiatry and Human Development, 6*, 26–32.

Chapter 15

Transsexualism and Choices

Thomas G. Webster

"I don't know what it means to be a woman. . . . I never use the word *woman* with relation to myself . . . I have avoided my body, tried to get acquainted with it, but absolutely hate it. . . . My main problem is I have difficulty getting close to people."

These are words of Jane (John) H, a female transsexual in her early 20s as she expresses her struggle with gender identity. She had been receiving testosterone treatment for 3 months from a private physician when she applied to the George Washington University Gender Identity Program for sex-reassignment surgery.

Jane had wrestled with her problem since early childhood. "In the first grade I liked school but was bored and disruptive. I had stomachaches," Jane told us.

> I played with boys . . . tag, wrestling, ball. . . . In the second and third grades I got a boy's hat and jacket, which I wore over the dress I had to wear to school. . . . My mother wanted me to play with girls, but I did not. . . . My grandmother is the main one in my early memories. She took care of us. . . . She loved sports. . . . I thought of myself as a boy, but there was nothing in my life to say it was true. My idol was Mickey Mantle. I switch-hit, but my neck was not thick enough.
>
> I first got depressed when I was in the eighth grade. . . . The only people I was interested in were girls, but I had to keep it hidden. . . . I loved gym, but got into trouble—I was so goddamn competitive. . . . I hated the locker room . . . was terribly ashamed of breast development, self-conscious, bent over . . . but I liked looking at other girls. Only one girl ever let me fondle her breasts. . . . I thought I was a lesbian, but a friend said, "Just a stage."
>
> From the seventh grade on I had a crush on a different girlfriend every year. I had a girlfriend in high school and college. Then she got pregnant and

Thomas G. Webster • George Washington University Medical Center, Washington, D.C. 20037.

> married the father. I was crushed. . . . My "female"-to-female relations were
> with older women—that is, no possibility of sex. . . . Now I relate mostly as
> a male.

Jane was grappling with intertwined biological, psychological, and social issues. The disharmony triggered a gender dysphoria syndrome of distress and strongly motivated Jane to have surgery "to become a complete man."

DEFINITION

Transsexualism is an extreme form of core gender identity reversal in which an anatomically normal person is aware of his/her biological sex but consistently feels himself/herself to be a member of the opposite sex. For example, a biologically female transsexual adolescent feels romantically and sexually attracted as a male to a "true and complete" female. Transsexuals sharply distinguish this yearning, at least by young adulthood, from a typical homosexual relationship.

KEY CONCEPTS

The issue of gender identity is universal. Development of identity is an essential process that evolves throughout childhood and adult life. The transsexual person's dramatic focus on body and gender accentuates to an uncommon degree the conflicts that we all experience to some extent in our development.

Although manifested mainly at the conscious subjective level as a "sense of identity," the development of identity is a conscious and unconscious process that requires integration of body image, physical and mental talents, personality and reaction traits, primary relationships, and finding one's place in society. Idealized fantasies and hopes may gradually give way to partial disillusionment, but opportunities and capabilities beyond earlier anticipations also come into play. A reasonably satisfactory resolution of identity conflicts is prerequisite for successful pursuit of adult intimacy, family life, and career satisfaction. The process is not rigid; rather, it is dynamic and developmental, with many individual variations and options.

The transsexual person's childhood confusion, distress, and social traumata evolve into identity problems of adolescence. Apparently these childhood determinants are crucial, but the adolescent phase of transsexual identity development is of key clinical importance. Transsexual persons often struggle to maintain a more total identity and self-esteem by attributing most of their problems to their misfit bodies. "I am a man in a woman's body," they will say. They perceive changing their bodies as the solution; all other issues seem to hinge on the surgical solution to an extremely complex internal and external reality problem. They usually do not seek medical or psychiatric help until they become adolescents or, most commonly, adults.

Experts have not yet been able to predict accurately which children, even highly effeminate boys and/or "masculine" girls, will later become transsexuals. In contrast, clinicians are usually able to make an accurate differential diagnosis when treating adolescents, and particularly adults, who have gender identity problems.

Frustrations, failures, and depression at any formative stage can undermine self-esteem and erode healthy identity development. During adolescence and young adulthood, gender identity and related emotional developmental tasks are commonly delayed until the individual feels desperate about the cumulative stress and strain. Despite recent trends toward earlier intervention, by the time many transsexuals do seek help, they view their adjustment problems primarily in terms of imagined surgical solutions.

With or without surgery, the long-range solution for the transsexual person requires patience, understanding, emotional support, experimentation, exploration—and more patience. The relative personal and cultural isolation of transsexuals accentuates their problems. Discovery of real options and limitations takes time, ingenuity, assistance, fortitude, and drive. Transsexual persons face problems and must make decisions through trial and error at every stage of their life adjustment.

EPIDEMIOLOGY

Cases of presumed transsexualism have been reported since ancient times and in a wide variety of primitive and modern cultures (Green & Money, 1969; Money, 1988). Studies in the United States have indicated that there are four times as many male as there are female transsexuals; a more recent study reported a male-to-female ratio of 2 to 1. (Schmidt, Halle, Lucas, & Meyer, 1980). Reliable epidemiologic data are still lacking; however, from available information, I would conservatively estimate a prevalence of 1 or 2 cases of transsexualism per 100,000 population, or from 2,000 to 5,000 cases in the United States. Differences in the strictness of applied diagnostic criteria add to the uncertainty of the data. Reported cases tend to be applicants for surgery. Many cases presumably go unreported, while others may be duplicates of individuals applying to more than one clinic. Age of first reported diagnosis ranges from 12 to 65, but the report most often occurs between the ages of 18 and 30. Cases of sex-change surgery were first reported in 1931 and later popularized by Christine Jorgensen's operation in Sweden in 1953. Initially performed mainly in Europe, the United States, and North Africa, and now in Asia and Australia, such operations now probably number over 2,000 worldwide. Many sex-change operations are not reported in scientific literature. Most reported series of cases are from university clinics, but many operations now are also being performed by other surgeons and are not so novel.

CLINICAL OBSERVATIONS

Case histories of transsexual individuals typically extend back to early childhood or earliest memory. The child feels a natural preference for the opposite gender role and behavior, which becomes a source of confusion and social problems. A firm sense of opposite gender identity usually crystallizes along with other identity issues during adolescence or young adulthood. These issues include other aspects of the person's self-image and his/her place in society, in work, and in relation to family, peers, and others. In our culture the cross-gender behavior of boys as compared with the behavior of tomboyish girls is generally more flagrant and troublesome to peers and concerned adults. Most effeminate boys and tomboyish girls do not become transsexuals, and predicting criteria are not yet clearly established. From at least the time of puberty, transsexuals are romantically attracted to persons of the same biological sex. In their own minds they are usually attracted, however, not a homosexuals but as members of the opposite sex. They find physical education classes and locker-room exposure to classmates agonizing and avoid them whenever possible. Adults and peers alike display their disapproval. Thus, the transsexual child or youth seeks and appreciates acceptance by friends or relatives.

Transsexuals usually regard their genitals with disinterest or disdain. Sexual impulses and overt behavior vary widely in different transsexuals, but transsexuals typically prefer to minimize stimulation of their genitals. Among biological males erection and climax are typically reduced; distinct exceptions should raise questions about the diagnosis of transsexuality.

During adolescence and young adulthood, recurrent conflicts and disappointments arise concerning work, social adjustment, and close relationships. Transsexuals often limit themselves to a constricted life-style or subculture. A code of one's own, sometimes shared with others in a transsexual and transvestite subculture, becomes essential for survival. Intense feelings, precipitated by traumatic experiences, are avoided only by living an extremely constricted and private life. The intense yearning to be a "total woman" or a "total man" comes to dominate other aspects of life.

Physical examination and laboratory test results are typically unremarkable and correspond to biological gender. Within these normal limits, there is a wide variation in manifestation of sexual hormones, such as hirsute characteristics of male transsexuals. Mental examination is marked by the many striking qualities of appearance and behavior that resemble the preferred gender.

The *apparent* gender of applicants for sex-change surgery is usually more ambiguous than in the most classical cases, and there are problems of differential diagnosis. Voice, which is consistent with biological gender, is usually not strongly male or female but is more apt to be noticed if other inconsistencies are evident. Under the influence of hormone therapy, the patient's appearance, mannerisms, voice, and breasts will correspond even more consistently with the chosen gender role, even if he/she is ambiguous in one or more of these secondary sex characteristics.

Other mental reactions and personality features are individualized and are not part of the transsexual syndrome. Signs of psychosis or organic brain syndrome are typically absent; however, when individuals with psychotic features apply for surgery they are excluded from consideration. Sociopathic and histrionic traits commonly occur among male transsexuals but are quite variable. The apparent sociopathic and borderline personality traits vary in nature and degree from basic personality traits to strongly situational adolescent or adult adjustment reactions. Brief depressive reactions and grief commonly occur in either male or female transsexuals, but their mood is usually either dysphoric or quite cheerful and socially pleasant. Theoretically, deeper and more chronic depression may be inferred from self-defeating behavior, problems with self-esteem, occasional self-mutilation (such as of genitals), and preoccupation with cosmetic surgery or multiple elective operations. Direct clinical signs of major depression, however, are infrequent but are more apt to be brought to psychiatric attention. Serious suicidal attempts are also infrequent, although suicidal thoughts are common. Cases of suicide have been reported, and the suicidal risk must always be considered in clinical assessment and care.

The preceding clinical description is based on consistent trends in reported studies as well as my own observations and selective judgment. It is consistent with reports of earlier authors such as Green and Money (1969), Meyer (1974), Money (1988), and Stoller (1968, 1976, 1985a and b) and is characteristic of the more typical and classical transsexual syndrome. My own observations are based on approximately 70 persons I have seen from 1972 to 1990 in the George Washington University Gender Identity Program. Practically all were applicants for hormone and surgical treatment. Only a few of these individuals followed through to meet our criteria for and to have sex-reassignment surgery (our criteria and procedures are similar to those at other university clinics). By shopping around, several other persons have subsequently had surgery elsewhere, usually owing to quicker action from some private surgeons who do not require comprehensive psychiatric evaluation and psychotherapy.

For all of the patients I have seen—ranging in age from 17 to 63—life has been filled with many painful and difficult choices. An important goal of the clinician and therapist is to help the patient distinguish areas of choice from areas of little or no choice. Ultimately, many of the choices become manifest in the ongoing behavior and reactions of the patient as he or she engages in longer-range treatment and life adjustment.

Cases of the classical transsexual syndrome, sometimes called primary or true transsexualism, are seen less often than are cases marked by varying degrees of classical features. The lesser degrees of classical transsexualism may blend with other conditions that, with advancing age, may come to resemble but will never fully duplicate classical transsexualism.

Criteria for adult transsexualism in the third edition (revised) of the American Psychiatric Association's *Diagnostic and Statistical Manual of Mental Disorders,* (1987) are less specific and restrictive than either the preceding clinical description or classical transsexualism. In particular, the DSM-III-R criteria lack the long duration and striking cross-gender qualities seen in more classical or primary transsexualism. DSM-III-R lists the following criteria for adult transsexualism (diagnostic code 302.50):

A. Persistent discomfort and sense of inappropriateness about one's assigned sex.
B. Persistent preoccupation for at least two years with getting rid of one's primary and secondary sex characteristics and acquiring the sex characteristics of the other sex.
C. The person has reached puberty.

Performance of transsexual patients on standard psychological examinations such as Rorschach, Draw-a-Person, Minnesota Multiphasic Personality Inventory, and self-concept tests has demonstrated one dominant finding: high femininity and low masculinity (defined by attitudes, interest, self-concept, role, and fantasy) among biological male transsexuals, and high masculinity with low femininity among female transsexuals. A strongly overcompensating mental process is indicated by the finding that the femininity score of male transsexuals is much higher than the normative median for heterosexual women, and the masculinity score of female transsexuals is higher than the normative median for heterosexual men. Both male and female transsexuals also score in the lowest fifth of normative distribution on tests of sex knowledge based on general information about sexual physiology and behavior. Other trends are less marked in frequency and degree, are more variable among different cases, and are less relevant for differential diagnosis of transsexualism. Mild depression and psychological (ego) constriction are often found but are by no means universal. Findings on other standard psychological test variables are individualized and usually within normal limits of deviation.

DIFFERENTIAL DIAGNOSIS

Differential diagnosis considerations include schizophrenia, organic brain disease, sociopathy, and transvestism. Differential diagnosis is clear when any of these conditions occur in pure or classic form. Mixtures and gradations make the task more difficult. For example, accentuated transsexual-like features may occur during periods of stress, developmental crises, or aging.

With more patients coming through the now more accessible clinics for transsexuals, there is a higher proportion of complicated and mixed cases. More public information and grapevine misinformation about transsexualism and sex-change surgery have led a greater variety of people to seek consultation for surgery for real or imagined transsexualism. Moreover, consultation and treatment resources are more widely available. Diagnostic criteria for transsexualism are now less strict compared with the more typical or classical transsexualism, with these less strict criteria made official by DSM-III in 1980, and remaining much the same in DSM-III-R in 1987. Also, greater varieties of treatment methods are offered, by more physicians, and by a widening circle of nonphysician service-market providers. All these trends have placed a greater burden on the physician with the task of making the differential diagnosis. Some clinics have become more strict in their application of criteria for surgery, even while diagnosing transsexualism more readily. Recent and future "breakthroughs" in new nonsurgical treatment methods for transsexualism should be evaluated in light of the widening door to diagnosis of transsexualism.

Under current conditions I have found it useful to make at least a gross distinction between classical or primary transsexualism on the one hand and delayed or secondary transsexualism on the other. Stoller (1968, 1976, 1982, 1985, 1985b), Person and Ovesey (1974a and b), and more recent authors have similarly used the terms *primary* and *secondary* *transsexualism* for similar distinctions. Both primary and secondary transsexualism may occur within the DSM-III-R diagnostic criteria and category (code 302.50) for transsexualism. DSM-III-R does not list subtypes of transsexualism.

Within a larger category of "Gender Identity Disorders," DSM-III-R lists three types:

1. Transsexualism (code 302.50)
2. Gender identity disorder of childhood (302.60)
3. Gender identity disorder of adolescence or adulthood, nontranssexual type (GIDAANT) or not otherwise specified (302.85)

Some cases of secondary transsexualism may cross the boundary between 302.85 and 302.50.

Classical or primary transsexualism is not always easy to distinguish, but it includes consistent cross-gender performance and behavior from early childhood and continues through adolescence and adult stages of identity. Mannerisms, appearance, and behavior are more typical—often strikingly so—of the preferred gender, and sexual attitudes and behavior are more typical of the primary transsexual syndrome.

Delayed or secondary transsexualism includes cases that are apt to have evidence of transvestism, common homosexuality, or sometimes homophobia. Rare cases of natural hormone-induced gender reversal (such as an anatomical female who reverses gender in adolescence with natural male levels of testosterone during adolescence and adulthood) are a form of biological intersex disorder and not technically transsexualism. Other delayed types of transsexualism may be described and clarified in the future.

Homophobic homosexuality can be particularly confusing because of the largely unconscious element. Some cases with homophobia can also meet DSM-III-R diagnostic criteria for transsexualism and are hence one type of delayed transsexualism. Other cases with homophobia have had overt homosexual experiences of the more common type, while most cases are primarily heterosexual in sexual performance and have gender identity consistent with biological gender.

Transvestism provides an important example of differential diagnosis in transsexualism of biological males. This is generally not a diagnostic problem in biological females, for whom transvestism is essentially unknown despite three interesting cases reported by Stoller (1985b). Classical transvestism, DSM-III-R code 302.30, with its fetishistic (erotic) cross-dressing, is not a differential diagnostic problem because the classical transvestite clearly views himself—and is viewed by others—as male. The main manifestation is not gender identity but sexual fetishism.

The Female Transsexual

In recent years, augmented by the women's movement, an increasing number of biological females have sought evaluation for surgical reassignment in gender identity clinics. In the largest study to date, Schmidt, Halle, Lucas, and Meyer (1980) at the Johns Hopkins University Medical Center reported on 132 biological females who had requested surgical reassignment from 1971 to 1978. They reported that this increase in female applicants caused a shift in the male–female ratio of their gender identity clinic from 4 : 1 to 2 : 1.

The Johns Hopkins female transsexual patients reported in this study differed as a group from the group of patients—predominantly male transsexuals—I have seen at the George Washington University Clinic and from other groups of predominantly male transsexuals as reported in other studies. Schmidt and associates applied the broader DSM-III criteria in their "primary diagnosis" of transsexualism and focused on the female transsexual. They also reported that in this group of female transsexuals—as compared with most studies of mainly male transsexuals—there was a preponderance of whites, a high incidence of reportedly happy childhoods, comparatively late onset of strong desire to be of the opposite gender, more stable job histories and primary relationships, and a lower incidence of sociopathy and histrionic traits.

The Schmidt et al. study illustrated that from a clinical perspective—contrary to a stereotyped view of transsexuals—there is a great variety of individual manifestations and, therefore, a great variety of potential choices open to transsexual persons.

Of the 132 female patients in the study (ranging in age from 12 to 58 years), 127 were diagnosed as transsexuals. Of these, 84% were single, 2% were married, and 14% were separated or divorced; half of the latter 16% had children.

As for the patients' sexual experiences, 56% had been exclusively homosexual, 34% had been bisexual, and 10% had had no sexual experience. The patients with no sexual experience tended to be very young or to have schizoid characteristics. Nearly all of the patients objected to being regarded as "homosexual" in the usual sense.

Fifty-three percent of the Schmidt et al. patients received no secondary psychiatric diagnosis. The others had moderate to moderately severe symptoms associated with a variety of neurotic and characterological disorders; e.g., 25 had a secondary diagnosis of depressive illness, 11 of borderline personality, 7 of adolescent adjustment reaction, 7 of passive-dependent personality, 5 of schizophrenia-paranoid type, 9 of other personality disorders (3 each of antisocial, inadequate, and hysterical personality), 3 of habitual excessive drinking, and 3 of obsessional neurosis. Recurrent suicidal ideation occurred among 13% of the 127 patients, and 16% reported suicide attempts.

Of these female transsexuals, 56% had been reared by both biological parents. In 36% of their homes the father had been absent, in 5% the mother had been absent, and in 4% both parents had been absent.

Sibling order was randomly distributed among the 91% who had siblings. Remembrances of family life were predominantly happy for 74% of the patients. The unhappy childhood family memories of the remaining 25% included parental fighting, parental drinking, and physical abuse of their mothers. Childhood tomboyish behavior was reported by 83% of the patients. Tomboyish behavior included preference for masculine dress, awareness of sexual feelings toward girls, preference for traditional male toys and play activities, and negative attitudes toward female pubertal development. Nine percent of the patients reported childhood cross-dressing without tomboyish behavior, and 8% had no memories of cross-gender behavior as children.

Only one of the 127 female transsexuals reported delayed menarche. Eight-four percent of the patients reported a negative reaction to menstruation; 82% reported a negative reaction to breast development. This finding, characteristic of female transsexualism, contrasts with the results of the Ehrhardt et al. 1979 study of lesbians cited by Schmidt et al. (1980). Ehrhardt et al. found that lesbians are not so apt to report negative reactions to the onset of menses or to pubertal development. In another study, Nachbahr (1977) found that female transsexuals had significantly more masculine gender role definitions than did comparison groups composed of either heterosexual or lesbian women.

Eight-five percent of the Schmidt et al. patients reported that they had not developed strong wishes to become men until they were 15 years of age or older. This correlates with my observation that despite the lifelong nature of transsexualism, identity development during adolescence and young adulthood crystallizes the problems for which the transsexual seeks medical help. As I have indicated, later onset of serious gender identity problems that receive a transsexual diagnosis is more common if one uses a broader definition of transsexualism.

In the Schmidt et al. study, 57% of the patients reported "a current love relationship with a female partner which had lasted one to five years. . . . The partners were described by patients as being feminine, maternal and domestic." The patients considered the term *homosexual* not applicable to these relationships and regarded biological males as competitors for their partners. "Every patient described their sexual activity with their current partner as satisfactory or good," wrote Schmidt. "They universally pointed out a feeling of incompleteness in their love making because they did not have a penis. Their current sexual fantasies were of being a man, making love to a feminine woman. In one-third of patients, sexual practices with the current partners involved mutual masturbation and oral-genital sex. The remainder of the group manually manipulated their partners but would not allow their own genitals to be touched. Although most of the patients expressed an interest in phalloplasty, only 5 used dildoes or other prosthetic devices during sexual activity."

Patients who reported no sexual experience and who often displayed schizoid traits expressed the hope that surgery would help them develop a better capacity to relate to others and thus to engage in sexual relations for the first time. According to Schmidt and associates, "Of the 95 patients in a current love relationship, 40% reported the relationship was stable. In 56% of the partnerships, the patient was concerned that her partner might leave her, citing the partner's concern about being involved in a homosexual relationship or occasionally the partner's interest in a biological male."

According to the patients' own reports, 38% of their partners, 32% of their parents, and 42% of their job supervisors or co-workers were informed and supportive of the patients' goals for surgical reassignment. In other cases these people were generally either neutral or not informed, though in 27% of the cases their parents who were informed opposed sex-change surgery.

"Despite being at the lower end of the socioeconomic scale, a finding in agreement with Pauly's (1974) study of 80 female transsexuals," wrote Schmidt and associates (1980), "these women have good work records and are contributing members of their community. . . . They move quietly into their cross-gender role within their communities, rarely calling attention to themselves." Ninety-five percent were employed (a much higher percentage than found in my series); their jobs were general clerical, skilled, or low-skilled positions. Most of the patients were high school graduates, and 75% were in the Hollingshead Social Class IV (low on a scale of I to V).

Female transsexuals are relatively stable, cooperative, and reliable. They frequently suffer from depression and other psychiatric symptoms, seek a surgical solution to problems in maintaining primary relations and resolving other stressful dilemmas, undergo situational adjustment conflicts, and are isolated by their social deviance. These factors make them candidates for help and support from psychotherapy.

FEMALE AND MALE TRANSSEXUALS COMPARED

Clinical reports and psychological examinations reveal intriguing differences, despite similarities, between male and female transsexuals. Psychological studies also show that transsexuals differ from lesbians and from other homosexual and heterosexual groups. Male and female transsexuals share a particularly strong and consistent commitment to their opposite-gender roles. Pauly (1974) described this as a characteristic in his study of 80 female transsexuals. Derogatis, Meyer, and

Boland (1981) confirmed this strong commitment in spite of the Schmidt et al. evidence that 34% of the female transsexuals in their study reported sexual activities with males. The persistent commitment is a classical finding of clinical and psychological studies and is used as a differential diagnostic and predictive criterion, particularly in the assessment problems with male transvestite-transsexual complexities. However, Derogatis et al. do not consider this unswerving commitment to be as dramatic with female as with male transsexuals.

Although Finney, Brandsome, Tondon, & Leimaistre (1975), Stoller (1976, 1982, 1985b), and many other clinicians, including myself, have observed a high incidence of hysterical (histrionic) personality among male transsexuals, Schmidt et al. (1980) found hysterical personality as a secondary diagnosis in only 3 of 127 female transsexual patients. The same higher incidence in male compared with female transsexuals is true of sociopathic traits, whether in basic personality structure or as a secondary reaction related to gender issues and efforts to obtain surgery. The histrionic and sociopathic traits of male transsexuals may influence their flamboyant, theatrical behavior and their exaggerated female posturing. Although female transsexuals are equally committed to changing their biological gender assignment and score twice as high on masculine psychological profile scales as do heterosexual men, they reportedly do not draw particular attention to themselves through male posturing or appearance. Frequently they pass for men in highly masculine occupations.

Comparable differences between male and female transsexuals are observed in associated signs of psychopathology. Derogatis et al. (1981) have reported that

> there seems to be more evidence of dramatic psychopathology among male transsexuals than among female transsexuals. . . . Our female transsexual sample revealed little noteworthy symptomatology, with a symptom profile that was almost entirely below one standard deviation above the mean for normative distribution. The negative affect total score is almost equivalent to that of the heterosexual comparison group and falls at the 50th percentile. . . . Positive affect does show a diminution among [female] transsexuals. . . . Vigor appears to be the least affected, with both joy and contentment showing more sizeable reductions . . . although they are unhappy, we do not see evidence of an impending emotional decompensation in the group.

Derogatis et al. (1981) further reported that male transsexuals, when compared with female transsexuals, manifested a more conservative or conventional sexual attitude posture according to attitude scales. I have found that the conventional sexual attitudes of male transsexuals occur despite their reported unconventional sexual experiences and their openness in describing sexual experiences and feelings. Presumably this paradox partly reflects the more intensive and somewhat open struggle that boys, especially effeminate boys, have in sexual and gender development. This is also consistent with the evidence that transsexualism carries more drastic repercussions for male than for female transsexuals. Female transsexuals demonstrate better adjustment in other aspects of their lives, such as greater success and stability in work, residence, and primary relationships. Thus, female transsexuals apparently do not have as much emotional need to maintain a conservative attitude posture in regard to their sexuality and sexual experiences as do male transsexuals. However, Derogatis et al. (1981) found that the patterns of reported sexual fantasies of both male and female transsexuals differed from those of heterosexual comparison groups. They also found that knowledge of basic sexual information was limited among male and female transsexuals, whose average scores were in the lowest fifth of normative distribution.

ETIOLOGY

The etiology of transsexualism remains undetermined. Its occurrence throughout history and in widely different cultures makes an organic-hormonal theory intriguing, despite the absence in clinical laboratory studies of detectable differences between transsexual patients and their normal biological counterparts. Extreme psychological deviancy in gender identity compared with relatively normal psychological profiles in other dimensions and the absence of consistently striking mother–infant or child–family patterns of deviance also raise more serious inferences of a biological basis. Despite the great quantity of scientific data on sex, hormones, behavior, and gender identity, as was detailed in the comprehensive 1978 Ciba Foundation Symposium report, no direct association was established between biological influences of the various developmental stages and the occurrence of the classical transsexual syndrome. Transsexualism does not follow a genetic pattern of distribution in reported clinical studies. Out of hundreds of reported cases, well-documented examples in which two transsexuals come from the same family are extraordinarily rare. Stoller (1982) reported one of the rare known cases; in that case two brothers were transsexual. This does not rule out the possibility of a genetic predisposing influence, but such an influence may require the presence of other factors. Sensitive to evidence of male bias, Fausto-Sterling (1985) reviewed research findings in her book about "the myths of gender":

> Clearly, in contrast to the body of work done on male development, the final word on the genetic control of female development has yet to be written. That it has not yet been fully researched is due both to technical difficulties

and to the willingness of researchers to accept at face value the idea of
passive female development . . . "testosterone equals male—absence of testosterone equals female." . . . If, however, one notes the pervasiveness
throughout all layers of our culture of the notion of "female as lack," then
one learns from this account that such rock-bottom cultural ideas can intrude
unnoticed even into the scientist's laboratory.

Her conclusions emphasized that "whichever direction of change [in the
development of gender identity] the human hallmark of enormous biological complexity and psychological flexibility shines through."

The most dramatic genetically related finding, involving the H-Y
antigen test in transsexuals, is relatively recent and still in the process of
research for confirmation and clarification. Eicher (a German gynecolog-
ist) et al. (1979) reported on 12 of 15 transsexual patients—later 57 of 61
patients, 33 males and 28 females—in whom the presence or absence of
H-Y antigen was unexpectedly abnormal, such as absent in transsexual
males when it would normally be expected to be present in males. The
H-Y antigen is found on the cell membrane of all male tissues, is considered an expression of a gene, is instrumental in testicular versus ovarian
development in utero, but apparently is not so directly involved during
subsequent stages of masculinization or feminization that depend on the
presence or absence of testosterone and other factors. Male transsexuals
have the expected 46 XY chromosomes of males, and female transsexuals have the expected 46 XX chromosomes of females, as summarized
by Pauly in Green and Money (1969). Transsexual males and females
have normal gonadal development (testes and ovaries, respectively) in
which the H-Y antigen must have been present or absent, respectively,
during early embryonic life. However, recent and ongoing research has
shown that a large number of XY (male) transsexuals do not react
positively to the H-Y antigen test, whereas XX (female) transsexuals do.
Eicher et al. (1981) reported that this paradoxical response was to be
found in 93% of all transsexuals (male and female) studied; Engel,
Pfafflin, and Wiedeking (1980) reported the same paradoxical response
in 65% of all transsexuals studied. These results from Germany are still
to be confirmed elsewhere, and the biological complexities are still being
unraveled by further research. Hoenig (1981) provided a review of the
subject from which the above information was freely drawn.

In animal experiments, prenatal administration of opposite-sex hormones can produce adult gender-reversed sexual behavior. Of course,
comparable experiments cannot be done with humans, and the active
study of human "experiments of nature" is still inconclusive and controversial. With monozygotic twins, for example, one twin might become
transsexual while the other develops as a heterosexual. A few cases of
gender reversal have been reported in which an individual was assumed

to be of one gender at birth but was later found to be congenitally hypogonadal and thus hormonally and psychologically of the opposite gender. This does not, however, explain the classical transsexual syndrome that involves no clear evidence of gonadal or hormonal abnormality. Subtle varieties of prenatal hormonal influences may conceivably combine with other factors to produce the transsexual syndrome. The hormonal factors may be more dominant in some cases and relatively insignificant in others.

Another perspective of family influences, or the lack thereof, in producing transsexualism is in the study of children reared by transsexual parents. Green (1978, 1987) has studied 37 children who were being reared either by male or female transsexual parents (16 children) or by female homosexuals (21 children). The 16 children reared by transsexual parents were either born to the transsexual while he or she was still living in the sex role designated at birth—before switching roles—or to a mother married to a female-to-male transsexual, who thus became the stepfather of the child. (Among the transsexual parents, there were seven male-to-female and nine female-to-male transsexuals.) Of these 37 children, the 13 older children who reported erotic fantasies or overt sexual behaviors were all heterosexually oriented and unremarkable in their appropriate and firmly established gender orientation.

Before turning further to parents and families as environmental influences on gender development, what is known about the adult outcome of feminine boys and tomboyish girls? Studies have been meager and of two general types: longitudinal studies beginning in childhood, and retrospective reports of transsexual, homosexual, and transvestite patients with heterosexual persons as comparison groups.

Green is still in the process of longitudinal studies of children with prominent cross-gender behaviors, some of whom have reached adolescence. Green did earlier pilot studies with Money (Green & Money, 1969) and then with Stoller (Green, 1987; Stoller, 1976, 1985b). In preliminary reports (Green, 1979) of 60 feminine boys, originally ages 4 to 11, Green and Stoller found that of 13 boys who had reached early to midadolescence, "50% of the boys who have fantasies that accompany masturbation or nocturnal emissions respond to homosexual fantasies," and most of these also had heterosexual fantasies. Apparently no recognizable cases of pretranssexualism had emerged, but all 50 boys were still at too young an age for transsexualism to be definitely established or to be absolutely ruled out.

Green (1985, 1987) later reported further follow-up on 78 boys who by then were presumably around ages 10 to 18 years. "One group consisted of 66 clinically-referred boys whose behaviors were consistent with the diagnosis of gender identity disorder of childhood [DSM-III-R

Code 302.60]. Another group served as controls and consisted of 56 volunteers selected on the basis of demographic matching. Two-thirds of each group were reevaluated for sexual orientations; 30 of the 44 who previously had shown extensive cross-gender behavior and none of the 34 in the comparison group were bisexually or homosexually oriented" (as compared with primarily heterosexually oriented). Apparently none of the 78 boys in this reevaluation—none from either group—had become transsexual, though most were still too young to be entirely sure.

Tomboyism in girls is more common than feminism in boys and more often converts to more conventional gender-appropriate behavior in adolescence. Green is conducting a large-scale developmental study of tomboys. In his preliminary report (Green, 1985), based on an earlier pilot sample, of four girls who were more tomboyish than typical tomboys and stated they wished they were boys, one was living as a young adult man and receiving male hormone treatment. Green later reported (Green, 1987) further follow-up studies on "sissy boys" as well as tomboyish girls.

Of retrospective studies, the report of Schmidt et al. (1980) on female transsexuals, including the patients' reports of childhood behavior, has been described earlier. Hellman, Green, Gray, and Williams reported a study (1981) of "homophobia" in 43 transsexuals, 78 homosexuals, and 43 heterosexuals, all of whom were adult biological males. This study included systematic data on the subjects' recall of childhood experiences and found that the transsexuals were significantly more apt, compared with homosexuals and heterosexuals, to report extensive cross-gender behavior during childhood. A transsexual outcome was "most reliably predicted" by recall of "Barbie-type doll play" (statistically significant compared with homosexuals, $\chi^2 = 27.64$, $p = .0001$) and of "helping mother with chores" ($\chi^2 = 9.04$, $p = 0.1$). Cross-gender peer group composition and a desire for female sexual anatomy during childhood also "appear to be important in differentiating the pre-transsexual from other groups." Hellman et al. found that male transsexuals who did not display extremely feminine traits as boys frequently developed homophobia as adults. "Although childhood religiosity (sometimes associated with homophobia) is not a predictor of transsexualism, it is a late determinant of attitudes and may function to maintain the established mode of sexual identity."

Stoller (1968, 1982, 1985b) has studied the psychodynamics of transsexual patients and their family and childrearing patterns. Although observing that the early developmental stages are critical in gender identity development, he noted the lack of sufficient basic and clinical research knowledge and that there is a great need for more extensive research before arriving at conclusions in theory and clinical practice. He has also pointed out the significant differences in male transsexual and female transsexual psychodynamics, particularly the more complicated task of gender identification for boys. A boy must normally make a psychological shift, including some rebellion and independence, to establish his identity as a male. This normal shift must occur after primary and formative experience with his mother, even though he must remain quite dependent on his mother during the process.

Stoller (1976, 1982, 1985b) noted there to be no clear and consistent patterns in the family interactions that distinguish the classical transsexual syndrome. However, Stoller has identified several trends concerning parents—particularly mothers—of pretranssexual boys, as compared with mothers of other effeminate boys and men. "The overprotectiveness that is often reported in homosexual men's mothers is given with more strings attached [more need to conform to the mother's control] than I find in these mothers [of transsexuals]," Stoller stated. "The latter have created for their infant sons a blissful closeness in which almost all wishes are granted. . . . Also, the mothers of transsexuals give less ambivalently to their sons as compared to the mothers of many homosexuals, mothers of transvestites, and mothers of other effeminate men." Stoller found that when the pretranssexual boys' mothers had been young girls, they were strikingly competitive with boys and often wore boys' clothing.

Stoller also pointed out the role of "powerful family dynamics" at crucial early stages in the development of transsexualism, and an "excessively close symbiosis between mother and infant" with the "father absent" either literally or emotionally. He stated that the pretranssexual infant's physical beauty, confirmed by other members of the family, often sparked the close attachment between mother and child. It is also Stoller's impression that the parents of transsexuals, compared with parents of homosexuals, strove harder to avoid separation and divorce when conflicts were severe.

Stoller reported cases in which an unusual degree of body contact occurred between the mother and the pretranssexual infant. I have found such evidence in two of my transsexual patients. One patient recalled nestling closely against his grandmother (the main nurturing figure) all night and every night from earliest memory into school-age years. In another case the mother told me she kept the baby in her lap or closely next to her in bed for many hours each night and in her arms much of the day during infancy.

Such a mother–infant relationship is consistent with theories of complications in earliest identity development and early individuation. Such histories, however, are not usually confirmed in most cases of transsexualism. By the time most transsexual patients see a psychiatrist for evaluation (usually for the avowed purpose of getting the necessary approval for sex-change surgery), details of very early events are not reliably or consistently established. Longitudinal studies from infancy to young adulthood would be useful, although it would be rare to identify pretranssexual individuals at such an early stage. Even the theoretical issues lack precision. Apparently the "symbiosis" of the mother and the pretranssexual infant, as postulated by Stoller, is more partial, specific, or benign than the symbiosis associated with childhood psychosis. Unfortunately, Stoller's theory does not explain how an influence so dramatic as a symbiotic mother–infant relationship—with the father "absent"—in one sector of infant development leaves other sectors so relatively normal. Nevertheless, the work of Stoller and Green with children and families is helping to elucidate the murky early psychological pathways of transsexual development. Somewhere they may find a common path with investigators who are exploring the equally murky biological territory.

The study of hermaphrodites and pseudohermaphrodites, individuals who have mixed or ambiguous biological gender, has been useful for distinguishing biological and childrearing factors in gender identity development. Most findings are consistent with child development knowledge, including psychoanalytic and psychodynamic knowledge of gender development. However, hormonal influences during prenatal and later stages can complicate and apparently override socioenvironmental childrearing influences.

From their review of studies of the influence of prenatal hormones on psychosexual development, Ehrhardt and Meyer-Bahlburg (Ciba Foundation Symposium, 1978) found evidence "for the powerful effects of early social environmental conditioning on gender identification." The authors held that "the evidence for such effects becomes even more persuasive when one considers the finding that hermaphrodite children—with both ambiguity of their sex organs at birth and subsequent exposure to confusion by pubertal hormones and secondary sex characteristics discordant with their sex of rearing—usually identify firmly with their assigned gender."

Stoller (1976) had earlier assessed several subjects with genital/ hormonal abnormalities who underwent a gender reversal. For example, a baby with female genitals was reared as a girl; no one realized the coexistence of male hormone levels that eventually predominated and presumably caused the gender reversal when this girl became a boy many years later.

Although these hormonal studies and cases did not deal directly with transsexualism, they made a significant contribution in regard to the interplay of biological, psychological, and social forces in different persons, families, and cultures and at different stages of gender identity development.

In summary, it appears likely that different combinations of genetic, biologic, psychologic, and family factors at prenatal, infant, early childhood, and adolescent stages of development are involved in the rare creation of a classical transsexual person. The H-R antigen test holds promise, but it is still very far from a simple routine blood or urine test, for diagnostic screening, such as is done for phenylketonuria in newborn infants.

TREATMENT

Treatment measures for transsexual patients include psychotherapy, hormone therapy, surgery, and environmental management. Some transsexuals also attend to their secondary sex characteristics with cosmetic grooming, hair removal, and training in voice, speech, posture, and movement. For the classical transsexuals, however, the chosen gender characteristics develop more naturally.

PSYCHOTHERAPY. Psychotherapy does not ordinarily change the gender identity of transsexual patients, particularly primary transsexuals. The recent increase of patients with more partial transsexual features, combined with DSM-III's broader definition of "transsexual," has been associated with better differential diagnosis of subtypes and more active psychotherapeutic efforts. There are now more frequent reports of reorientation of patients, usually to homosexuality, sometimes to heterosexuality, and often to roles more consistent with biological gender identity.

Several types of psychotherapy can be important for longer-range life adjustment and developmental adaptation, particularly at times of acute life crises and transitions. Patients seeking surgery often have a history of ever-worsening crises and symptoms, with progressively narrowing alternatives; they finally find greater peace of mind through a decision to become more "complete" through surgery. They dream of the day when they might have a more permanent partner, a more secure job, and a greater sense of self-esteem and fulfillment through a surgical solution. The potentially useful therapies include specific symptomatic individual or group psychotherapy, behavior therapy, and family or couples therapy, sometimes combined with temporary use of psychotropic medication for relief of disabling symptoms. Patients are more apt to be motivated for psychiatric help in episodes of distress, which the therapist can use to foster a therapeutic alliance and orientation to recurrent and longer-range issues.

The use of psychotherapy in transsexualism frequently faces difficult obstacles. Transiency and infrequent contacts seriously impair psychotherapeutic efforts, as does the common "benign sociopathic" quality of the male transsexual's relations with the therapist, as mentioned previously in this chapter and by Stoller (1976). The long experience of internal psychological conflict and disharmony with external realities usually leaves transsexual patients with an underlying hopelessness by adulthood; they often despair of finding a solution within themselves. Their motivation for psychotherapy is often low, though apparently less low for female transsexuals (Schmidt et al., 1980). A major task of the psychiatrist, then, is to use consultations and other contacts to foster awareness of potential psychotherapeutic tasks and adaptive alternatives. The work must be oriented to current and future realities, clarifying the mixture of gender identity issues and choices for that individual, and finding new feasible solutions.

Problems in attempts to use psychotherapy or psychoanalysis to change gender identity in transsexuals are linked to the nature of the condition, the limitations of these methods, and the characterological and motivational problems of the patients. In reports from private practitioners and therapists at gender identity clinics and in my own experience, only a small minority of patients are introspectively or psychologically minded while also possessing the ego strength, the capacity for a deeply therapeutic relationship, and/or the motivation and financing to pursue psychoanalysis or long-term insight therapy.

The trust and reliance that keep other types of chronic or long-term medical and psychiatric patients in periodic contact with a physician or therapist are apparently not so common in gender identity patients. Often the first psychiatric contact is a required routine after deciding to apply for surgery. During the months and years required for fulfilling criteria for surgery, while they are uncertain of being "approved" for surgery, patients have some natural distrust of the doctors who do not rapidly give that desired assurance. Such patients tend to shop around or return sporadically. For operated patients who have found such acceptance and approval, some become polysurgery addicts in pursuing a sequence of additional operations, and some see hormones as the only continuing treatment needed from doctors. Such patients tend to leave untapped the potential usefulness of psychotherapy for other symptoms and for the crucial problems of longer-range adolescent and adult development and life adjustment.

I have made some progress in establishing therapeutic alliance for nonsurgical issues with about 20% of my transsexual patients. Other significant deterrents have been low income, variable employment, and lack of insurance coverage for outpatient psychiatry. The patients who return, whether regularly or infrequently, usually have more stable employment histories, which reflects their personal strengths as well as their financial security. My experience is not necessarily typical of that at all clinics. At other clinics the financial feasibility of psychotherapy—for both therapist and patient—may not be such a barrier, and there are different assortments in the characteristics of patients that apply in different clinics at different times. The more stable history of employment and primary relationships and the lack of sociopathic qualities in female transsexual patients would appear to make them better candidates for psychotherapy than their male counterparts. For males and females few reports and data are available, however, regarding what type of psychotherapy, consultation, and/or counseling has been done, how financed, and by which type of therapist. It is difficult to assess how effectively clinics use surgery consultations and symptomatic crises to foster a therapeutic alliance with the same therapist on longer-range and recurrent adult development issues that plague many transsexuals over the years, regardless of whether or not they have surgery.

Barlow, Abel, and Blanchard (1979) have reported a singular but significant behavior therapy program that successfully changed gender-related behavior in three young male transsexual patients. A systematic sequence of intensive behavior modification procedures were done, first on a 17-year-old. The follow-up report described no reversal of the gender identity changes that occurred with treatment of these three patients. The first patient, after 6½ years, described himself as "completely sexually reoriented." The second and third patients, who were somewhat older, had retained their new male gender identity, reported no desire for sex-change surgery, and preferred to live as male homosexuals. Two of the patients were reportedly happy and had a reasonably good social adjustment; at last report, the third patient's "general functioning had deteriorated." To my knowledge, Barlow's methods and results have not yet been duplicated elsewhere.

As with other conditions, caution is needed regarding simpler psychotherapy interventions solely on the basis of symptoms as compared with therapy based on skilled understanding of the total person and longer-range issues. For example, one therapist's behavioral approach was to recommend that the new wife of a transvestite (a widower and father of two children) should sexually and seductively "reinforce his masculinity." Her efforts led to a state of panic in her husband that resulted in his mental hospitalization. He then further surrendered his previously successful, although troubled, male identity, divorced her, and became a transsexual woman.

HORMONE THERAPY. A reversible intermediate step short of irreversible surgery is provided by hormone therapy. The indications for hormone therapy are similar to those for surgery, although they become evident at an earlier phase. Physical and psychological changes produced by hormone therapy are less extreme than those produced by surgery, but hormone-induced changes are more systemic and visible to others. Voice, hair, breasts, body contours, genital physiology, and some emotional states are affected.

The decision to take hormones—with physician concurrence—and the resulting biological changes strongly reinforce a person's choices along an irreversible path. Relatively few transsexual patients decide to reverse direction after hormone therapy. However, erratic use over months and years, availability from private practitioners reported over transsexual-transvestite grapevines, and loose experimentation make the use of hormones among transsexuals less controlled and more difficult to study than is desirable at our current stage of medical knowledge. For physiological and psychological reasons, hormone therapy is a prerequisite to sex-reassignment surgery. Theoretically, just as diabetics take insulin, transsexuals take hormones indefinitely. Often, however, they do not follow a hormone regimen as religiously as diabetics with insulin, partly because of the lack of immediate or serious consequences of hormone lapse. The expense is prohibitive for some unemployed transsexuals, and thus their treatment may become more erratic. A useful secondary effect is that hormone therapy provides sustained, if intermittent, contact with a physician. This fact has not been sufficiently exploited as a means of fostering a modified but more active psychotherapeutic alliance.

ASSOCIATED PROCEDURES AND CHOICES. Change in secondary sexual characteristics, with or without hormones, may be augmented by training in voice, speech, and language (Walters & Ross, 1986), in body movements, and in gender-appropriate mannerisms and culture. Hair removal by electrolysis is common among male-to-female transsexuals. Additional decisions and choices include a variety of legal issues (such as name change, licenses, official documents, potential lawsuits) and ethical issues (irreversible decisions, manipulations, do good vs. do no harm, rights of patients, spouses, and employers).

SURGERY. Criteria for sex-change surgery have been presented in many reports. The George Washington University Gender Identity Program uses the following criteria, which are more strict and less inclusive than the APA's DSM-III-R criteria for diagnosis of transsexualism.

1. Patient has a lifelong history (from early childhood, usually before age 5) of regarding self or preferring role more like member of opposite gender than own gender—e.g., feeling like "a woman in a man's body."

2. Patient expresses dislike for own sexual organs, strong and consistent desire to have those of opposite sex.

3. Male transsexual has little genital response or interest in own genitals associated with sexual experience—e.g., little or no erection or interest in having penis stimulated. Female transsexual usually prefers to stimulate partner more than vice versa, often preferring to avoid stimulation of own breasts or genitals.

4. Psychiatric and psychological examinations have established transsexual diagnosis and ruled out psychosis, homosexuality, and transvestism (or fetishistic cross-dressing).

5. Physical exam and laboratory studies have established that patient is a biologically normal male or female.

6. Patient has been on hormone therapy for at least 1 year.

7. Patient has lived and worked successfully as adult in chosen gender role for at least 1 year.

8. Patient has availed himself/herself of some form of psychotherapy for at least 1 year.

9. Patient has notified parents, next of kin, or significant family member. Family member has been interviewed by psychiatrist of gender identity team.

10. Patient has made financial arrangements to cover the entire cost of the preliminary assessment and care, surgery, hospitalization, and immediate follow-up, and has retained an attorney to counsel and to witness the signing of the surgery consent papers.

11. Patient has demonstrated strong and consistent drive for surgery over a number of years (at least 2 years, usually longer) and in spite of obstacles.

12. Interdisciplinary gender identity team has met to review case and decide whether criteria have been met satisfactorily, and have agreed to a decision for surgery. Diagnosis, psychosocial readiness, and timing of surgery primarily are psychiatric decisions; biological and endocrinological readiness is primarily a surgical and/or gynecological decision. Surgery date set at least 1 to 2 months in advance, with intervening intensified individual psychotherapy and some form of family therapy. Patient should demonstrate evidence of commitment to surgical and psychiatric follow-up care.

Much of the surgery in this country and elsewhere is performed by private surgeons rather than by surgeons working in university medical centers that have gender identity programs. These private surgeons usually request that the patient obtain a letter regarding diagnosis from a psychiatrist or psychologist. A few such patients have come to consultation sessions expecting to be given such a letter after only one interview, then felt frustrated by our more conservative approach. Many apparently obtain such a letter from sources unknown to me.

In our clinic most applicants drop out not because they fail to meet the essential diagnostic criteria, but because they fail to pursue the espoused surgery objective with the required patience and persistence. The financial hurdle, too, is very significant; the cost of surgery is beyond the means of many of my patients, particularly given the problems manifest in their job histories. Mild degrees of sociopathic type traits are apt to become exaggerated in response to the stress of this externally imposed limit. The patients' self-defeating and ineffectual adaptive abilities may all become more evident; they may drop out of the program without explanation. Patients who drop out lose other medical, psychotherapeutic, and social assistance and may once again become isolated from a potential support system.

Presumably, a significant number pursue and may find solutions, including surgery, in other cities or clinics; however, I have only rare reports of such outcomes. I have had more occasion to hear from patients—sporadically, often with several years intervening—who are apt to give financial reasons for not yet fulfilling their persistent hope for surgical intervention and for dropping out of contact with me and the Gender Identity Program.

An individual who pursues the Gender Identity Program and meets the surgical criteria may achieve considerable personal growth, at least when intensive psychotherapy and family therapy occur during the pre- and postsurgery phases. For example, one of my patients accomplished much more through psychotherapy during the last 3 months before surgery than during the previous several years of more sporadic visits. In joint sessions with next of kin, as well as in individual sessions, we dealt with emotionally charged issues, family myths, and the patient's personal distancing that had evolved since childhood. The patient's self-image, self-esteem, and anatomic fantasies were more emotionally charged, more accessible, and more effectively dealt with in psychotherapy.

After surgery the patient made a more complete and successful shift in work, career, neighborhood, and church associations, as well as in lasting intimate relations, than is usually reported. The expressed sense of "a new life" occurred simultaneously with the patient's reported sense of surprise shortly after surgery that "I'm still just the same person, even feels like the same body, not all so different as I expected— sort of a letdown in a way, but I feel just great." This mood persisted, in less dramatic form, during the 3 years of follow-up contact and successful postoperative life adaptation—in contrast to the patient's increasing hopelessness and depressive symptoms during the 5 years before surgery.

Follow-Up

Meyer and Reter (1979) provided a valuable review of six U.S. follow-up studies of transsexuals who had undergone sex-change surgery from 1965 to 1975. They also reported their own follow-up study, completed in 1974, of 50 applicants for surgery at the Johns Hopkins University—the first follow-up to comprise both patients who had undergone surgery and patients who had not. "None of the operated patients voiced regrets at reassignment, the operative loss of reproductive organs, or the substitution of opposite sex facsimiles (though one female transsexual requested removal of a phallus after many surgical complications)." The "unoperated subjects made more use of psychiatric contacts both before and after the initial interview, which relates to their somewhat higher educational level and the recent greater emphasis on psychiatric screening [by the clinic]. Additionally, these patients, being unoperated, continued to seek various psychiatric endorsements for their quests: 40% subsequently had surgery; 14% gave up all active pursuit [of sex reassignment surgery]" (Meyer & Reter, 1979).

The initial Meyer and Reter (1979) study concentrated on the more observable criteria of adaptation, such as rating scales as to residence, education, socioeconomic status, job, cohabitation, and psychiatric contacts (the last being used only as an indicator of poor adjustment in this particular project) to arrive at an "adjustment score."

> Initial adjustment scores indicate that the original operated group was slightly more distressed [had lower initial scores] than the unoperated. Poorest follow-up scores occurred among a subgroup of patients originally unoperated who, during the follow-up period, precipitously had surgery elsewhere. Significant positive change in adjustment scores occurred over time for both the operated and unoperated patients.
>
> Although other constructions are possible, the most conservative interpretation of the data is that among the applicants for sex reassignment, there are operationally two groups who, in the face of a trial period, will self-select for or against surgery and that, in either instance, improvement will be demonstrated over time, as judged by observable behavioral variables. Sex reassignment surgery confers no objective advantage in terms of social rehabilitation [based on authors' rating system and statistical blends], although it remains subjectively satisfying to those who have rigorously pursued a trial period and who have undergone it. (Meyer & Reter, 1979)

Walters and Ross (1986) reported on postsurgery follow-up on 56 of the 68 male-to-female operated cases, 1976–1982, in Australia: "Approximately 80 percent of our patients reported good or satisfactory outcome after surgery, despite the fact that the vagina was deemed of inadequate dimensions (with pain and discomfort during intercourse) in 35 percent of them." For female-to-male reassignment surgery, mastectomy, hysterectomy, and bilateralsalipingo-oophorectomy are standard procedures with relatively little complication, but phalloplasty (construction of a penis) is universally problematic and often avoided in favor of a prosthesis. Walters and Ross reported one suicide among their postoperative cases. The patient had stated that she had no regrets about having had the operation; the suicide appeared to be related to the loss of her job, boyfriend, and self-esteem.

On the basis of the sufficiently positive postoperative outcomes evident from his review in 1981 of eight studies, Pauly (1981) questioned the decision of the Johns Hopkins program to discontinue sex-change surgery—given the knowledge that the Hopkins decision was based in part on the Meyer and Reter (1979) study and conclusions. Pauly's conclusions did not differ particularly from Meyer and Reter's about the great preponderance of satisfactory outcomes from surgery, but the reports Pauly reviewed did not include follow-up study of unoperated cases. Critiques by other authors of the Meyer and Reter methods and conclusions and the apparent consequences in terminating sex-change surgery at Johns Hopkins University Medical Center were more recently summarized by Stoller (1982).

Pauly's opinion concurs with my own and with the authors cited by Stoller. "The fact that this [Meyer and Reter] unoperated group showed significant positive change in adjustment is interesting, but hardly justifies the conclusion that surgery is not indicated for any applicants." In my opinion, the Meyer and Reter study of unoperated applicants for surgery was timely and significant. However, their study methods and conclusions were based on gross statistical groupings that by necessity obscured other differences in the operated and unoperated patients and obscured significant data used for clinical decisions based on more total assessment of each individual case at a given point in the transsexual person's individual development and the historical state of the field.

Despite his encouraging estimate of the value of surgery, Pauly cited risks and emphasized careful selection and alternative approaches. He emphasized that some investigators have estimated that up to 35% of transsexuals are "self-stigmatized, homophobic homosexuals," who should be helped with therapy to accept their homosexuality. He also discussed studies conducted in 1978 and 1980 that reported some success with nonsurgical adaptive solutions to the problems of such homosexuals and other gender-dysphoria patients (Pauly, 1981).

Follow-up studies indicate the value of careful psychiatric screening, rigorous application of trial periods before surgery, and systematic approaches that would base the choice of surgery on behavior observed over a longer period of time as well as the initial stated intent and ongoing choices of the patients.

There is a dearth of information about efforts made to convert the patients' surgery motivation into a longer-range therapeutic alliance that would help with specific issues of life adjustment and development. Stoller (1976, 1982, 1985b) described his variable psychoanalytic and psychotherapeutic experiences with selected transsexual patients and/or members of their families, but without context data about other transsexual patients in his institution's total pool of applicants. Meyer and Reter (1979) reported that "no attempt was made to habilitate unoperated patients in the cross-gender role. The patients were seen infrequently, given hormones, and were not urged or instructed in either direction. The program is interested, concerned, but noninterventive, recognizing the strength of the wish for sex reassignment, but adopting a position of watchful waiting with regard to it." However, Lothstein and Levine (1981, 1982) reviewed transsexual psychotherapy reports and their own active psychotherapy program at Case-Western Reserve University. They found that 70% of 50 "gender dysphoric patients . . . have adjusted to non-surgical solutions. . . . The crux of psychotherapy is establishing a therapeutic alliance."

These follow-up and psychotherapy studies reflect an encouraging increase in research and treatment activity oriented to long-range development and life adjustment that will, one hopes, provide improved outcomes in future treatment, prevention, and follow-up. If they are to help transsexual persons, professionals must not become overly preoccupied with hormone treatment and surgery, even while prescribing them.

CHOICES AND IMPLICATIONS

The choices available to transsexuals may be viewed differently by professionals, family members, the public, and transsexuals themselves. One problem is that choices usually seem more varied, easy, or obvious to the public, and often to health professionals, than they do to transsexual individuals. An equally significant problem for those working in the field is that the options are greater—not necessarily gender identity choice—at earlier stages of the transsexual's life than they are by the time the person seeks psychiatric help. Fortunately, because of greater media coverage and professional attention recently given transsexualism and other gender identity problems, an increasing number of transsexuals are now receiving attention at an earlier age. This allows professionals, families, and the patients themselves to aid more effectively the overall development and life adjustment of transsexual persons.

A dubious benefit of greater public acceptance of transsexualism and sex-change surgery, however, is that physicians may provide hormones and surgery under relatively uncontrolled circumstances for a condition that is still in experimental phases of treatment and research. Thus, the health system reinforces paradoxically the transsexual person's narrowed choice of hormones and surgery as *the* solution. Individual physicians may treat the transsexual with hormones and surgery but neglect the patient's other needs and potential choices, even though at least a letter from a psychiatrist or psychologist confirming the diagnosis prior to surgery is now fairly routine practice among surgeons in the United States. One can empathize with the patient's distress and difficult problems and with the physician's desire to help. However, the clinical field is currently marked by the same chaos that characterizes the lives of many transsexuals.

Transsexualism and sex-reassignment surgery tend to evoke attitudes and feelings that are based on universal human experience with male-female identity and sexual life. A veneer of "understanding" and acceptance sometimes obscures the deeper but natural discomfort evoked when one is in the presence of a transsexual person. Nevertheless, the underlying discomfort can manifest itself through various attitudes and behavior that adversely affect transsexuals and those who care for them. Emotional and conceptual learning tasks are required before therapists can feel and function at ease with persons who have this condition.

When working with transsexual persons, I have had to examine my own inner reactions over and over again, and I appreciated my patients' helping me to understand their experiences. Despite their strong tendency to regard a psychiatrist primarily as a judge who has the authority to grant or deny surgery, some have been able to work with me sufficiently to improve my capacity to work with them.

Transsexualism is not a whim. For the patient, sex-change surgery is far more than "cosmetic" surgery (as it is still classified by many insurance companies). The transsexual is a person with a special handicap who tries in a variety of ways to develop and adapt. In this difficult task, some apparent options turn out to be myths, and many real options are too seldom pursued. Too often transsexual persons become caught in the vicious circles of their own confused identity and of the confusing world in which they live.

References

American Psychiatric Association. (1987). *Diagnostic and statistical manual of mental disorders* (3rd ed., rev.). Washington, DC: Author.

Barlow, D. H., Abel, G. G., & Blanchard, E. B. (1979). Gender identity change in transsexuals. *Archives of General Psychiatry, 36,* 1001–1007.`

Ciba Foundation Symposium 69. (1978). *Sex, hormones and behavior.* New York: Elsevier-North Holland.

Derogatis, L. B., Meyer, J. K., & Boland, P. (1981). A psychological profile of the transsexual, II. The female. *Journal of Nervous and Mental Disease, 169,* 157–168.

Eicher, W., Spoljar, M., Cleve, H., Murken, J. D., Richter, K., & Stengel-Rutkowski, S. (1979). H-Y antigen in transsexuality. *Lancet, 2,* 1137–1138.

Eicher, W., Spoljar, M., Cleve, H., Murken, J. D., Richter, K., & Stengel-Rutkowski, S. (1981). Transsexuality and H-Y antigen. *Fortschritte der Medizin, 99,* 9–12.

Engel, W., Pfafflin, F., & Wiedeking, C. (1980). H-Y antigen in transsexuality and how to explain testis differentiation in H-Y negative males and ovary differentiation in H-Y antigen positive females. *Human Genetics, 55,* 315–319.

Fausto-Sterling, A. (1985). *Myths of gender: Biological theories about women and men.* New York: Basic Books.

Finney, J. C., Brandsome, J. M., Tondon, M., & Leimaistre, G. A., (1975). A study of transsexuals seeking gender reassignment. *American Journal of Psychiatry, 132,* 962–964.

Green, R. (1978). Sexual identity of 37 children raised by homosexual or transsexual parents. *American Journal of Psychiatry, 135,* 692–697.

Green, R. (1979). Childhood cross-gender behavior and subsequent sexual preference. *American Journal of Psychiatry, 136,* 106–108.

Green, R. (1985). Gender identity in childhood and later sexual orientation: Follow-up of seventy-eight males. *American Journal of Psychiatry, 141,* 339–341.

Green, R. (1987). *"Sissy boy syndrome" and the development of homosexuality.* New Haven: Yale University Press.

Green, R., & Money, J. (Eds.). (1969). *Transsexualism and sex reassignment* (pp. 235–242). Baltimore: Johns Hopkins Press.

Hellman, R. E., Green, R., Gray, J. L., & Williams, K. (1981). Childhood sexual identity, childhood religiosity, and "homophobia" as influences in the development of transsexualism, homosexuality, and heterosexuality. *Archives of General Psychiatry, 38,* 910–915.

Hoenig, J. (1981). Etiological research in transsexuals. *Psychiatric Journal of the University of Ottawa, 6,* 184–189.

Lothstein, I. M. (1982). Sex reassignment surgery: Historical, bioethical and theoretical issues. *American Journal of Psychiatry, 139,* 417–26.

Lothstein, I. M., & Levine, S. B. (1981). Expressive psychotherapy with gender dysphoric patients. *Archives of General Psychiatry, 38,* 924–929.

Meyer, J. K. (1974). Clinical variants among applicants for sex reassignment. *Archives of Sexual Behavior, 3,* 527–558.

Meyer, J. K., & Reter, D. J. (1979). Sex reassignment: Follow-up. *Archives of General Psychiatry, 36,* 1010–1015.

Money, J. (1988). *Gay, straight and in-between: The sexology of erotic orientation.* New York: Oxford University Press.

Nachbahr, G. M. (1977). Gender role and sexuality in transsexual women as compared to homosexual and heterosexual women. *Dissertation Abstracts International, 38,* 1412–1413.

Pauly, I. B. (1974). Female transsexualism: II. *Archives of Sexual Behavior, 3*(6), 509–526.

Pauly, I. B. (1981). Outcome of sex reassignment surgery for transsexuals. *Australian and New Zealand Journal of Psychiatry, 15,* 45–51.

Person, E., & Ovesay, L. (1974a). The transsexual syndrome in males: I. Primary transsexualism. *American Journal of Psychotherapy, 28*(1), 4–20.

Person, E., & Ovesey, L. (1974b). The transsexual syndrome in males: II. Secondary transsexualism. *American Journal of Psychotherapy, 28*(2), 174–93.

Schmidt, C. W., Halle, E., Lucas, M. J., & Meyer, J. K. (1980, May). *Female transsexualism.* Paper presented at the annual meeting of the American Psychiatric Association, San Francisco.

Stoller, R. J. (1968). *Sex and gender: The transsexual experiment.* New York: Science House.

Stoller, R. J. (1976). *Sex and gender, II: The transsexual experiment.* New York: Aronson.

Stoller, R. J. (1982). Near miss: "Sex change" treatment and its evaluation. In M. F. Zales (Ed.), *Eating, sleeping and sexuality; Recent advances in basic life functions* (pp. 258–283). New York: Brunner/Mazel.

Stoller, R. J. (1985a). *Observing the erotic imagination.* New Haven: Yale University Press.

Stoller, R. J. (1985b). *Presentations of gender.* New Haven: Yale University Press.

Walters, W. A., & Ross, M. W. (Eds.). (1986). *Transsexualism and sex reassignment.* Melbourne: Oxford University Press.

Index